Techniques for Hair Restoration

Editors

LISA E. ISHII

LINDA N. LEE

FACIAL PLASTIC SURGERY CLINICS OF NORTH AMERICA

www.facialplastic.theclinics.com

Consulting Editor
J. REGAN THOMAS

May 2020 • Volume 28 • Number 2

ELSEVIER

1600 John F. Kennedy Boulevard • Suite 1800 • Philadelphia, Pennsylvania, 19103-2899

http://www.theclinics.com

FACIAL PLASTIC SURGERY CLINICS OF NORTH AMERICA Volume 28, Number 2
May 2020 ISSN 1064-7406, ISBN-13: 978-0-323-69594-7

Editor: Stacy Eastman
Developmental Editor: Laura Fisher

Facial Plastic Surgery Clinics of North America (ISSN 1064-7406) is published quarterly by Elsevier Inc., 360 Park Avenue South, New York, NY 10010-1710. Months of issue are February, May, August, and November. Business and Editorial Offices: 1600 John F. Kennedy Blvd., Suite 1800, Philadelphia, PA 19103-2899. Periodicals postage paid at New York, NY, and additional mailing offices. Subscription prices are $408.00 per year (US individuals), $692.00 per year (US institutions), $454.00 per year (Canadian individuals), $861.00 per year (Canadian institutions), $535.00 per year (foreign individuals), $861.00 per year (foreign institutions), $100.00 per year (US students), $100.00 per year (Canadian students), and $255.00 per year (foreign students). Foreign air speed delivery is included in all *Clinics* subscription prices. All prices are subject to change without notice. POSTMASTER: Send address changes to *Facial Plastic Surgery Clinics*, Elsevier Health Sciences Division, Subscription Customer Service, 3251 Riverport Lane, Maryland Heights, MO 63043. **Customer service: 1-800-654-2452 (US and Canada); 1-314-447-8871 (outside US and Canada); Fax: 314-447-8029; E-mail: journalscustomerservice-usa@elsevier.com (for print support); journalsonlinesupport-usa@elsevier.com (for online support).**

Reprints. For copies of 100 or more of articles in this publication, please contact the Commercial Reprints Department, Elsevier Inc., 360 Park Avenue South, New York, NY 10010-1710. Tel.: 212-633-3874; Fax: 212-633-3820; E-mail: reprints@elsevier.com.

Facial Plastic Surgery Clinics of North America is covered in *MEDLINE/PubMed* (*Index Medicus*).

Contributors

CONSULTING EDITOR

J. REGAN THOMAS, MD
Professor, Facial Plastic and Reconstructive
Surgery, Department of Otolaryngology–Head
and Neck Surgery, Northwestern University
Feinberg School of Medicine, Chicago, Illinois,
USA

EDITORS

LISA E. ISHII, MD, MHS
Associate Professor of Otolaryngology,
Department of Otolaryngology–Head and Neck
Surgery, Johns Hopkins School of Medicine,
Johns Hopkins Outpatient Center, Johns
Hopkins University, Baltimore, Maryland, USA

LINDA N. LEE, MD, FACS
Division of Facial Plastic And Reconstructive
Surgery, Assistant Professor, Department of
Otolaryngology–Head and Neck Surgery,
Harvard Medical School, Massachusetts Eye
and Ear, Associate Chief of Plastic Surgery,
Harvard Vanguard Medical Associates,
Boston, Massachusetts, USA

AUTHORS

MARC R. AVRAM, MD
Clinical Professor of Dermatology, Weill Cornell
Medical School, Private Practice, New York,
New York, USA

ANTHONY BARED, MD, FACS
Private Practice, Miami, Florida, USA

JENNY X. CHEN, MD
Resident, Department of Otolaryngology–Head
and Neck Surgery, Harvard Medical School,
Massachusetts Eye and Ear, Boston,
Massachusetts, USA

ADEEB DERAKHSHAN, MD
Resident, Department of Otolaryngology–Head
and Neck Surgery, Harvard Medical School,
Massachusetts Eye and Ear, Boston,
Massachusetts, USA

GORANA KUKA EPSTEIN, MD
Dr. Phillip Frost Department of Dermatology
and Cosmetic Surgery, University of Miami,

Foundation for Hair Restoration, Miami,
Florida, USA

JEFFREY EPSTEIN, MD, FACS
Dr. Phillip Frost Department of Dermatology
and Cosmetic Surgery, Foundation for Hair
Restoration, Department of Otolaryngology,
University of Miami, Miami, Florida,
USA

LISA E. ISHII, MD, MHS
Associate Professor of Otolaryngology,
Department of Otolaryngology–Head and Neck
Surgery, Johns Hopkins School of Medicine,
Johns Hopkins Outpatient Center, Johns
Hopkins University, Baltimore, Maryland,
USA

NATALIE JUSTICZ, MD
Resident, Department of Otolaryngology–Head
and Neck Surgery, Harvard Medical School,
Massachusetts Eye and Ear, Boston,
Massachusetts, USA

AMIT KOCHHAR, MD
Clinical Assistant Professor, Tina and Rick
Caruso Department of Otolaryngology–Head
and Neck Surgery, Keck School of Medicine of
USC, Los Angeles, California, USA

ANISHA R. KUMAR, MD
Department of Otolaryngology–Head and Neck
Surgery, Johns Hopkins School of Medicine,
Johns Hopkins Outpatient Center, Johns
Hopkins University, Baltimore, Maryland,
USA

SAMUEL M. LAM, MD, FACS, FISHRS
Private Practice, Lam Institute for Hair
Restoration, Plano, Texas, USA

LINDA N. LEE, MD, FACS
Division of Facial Plastic and Reconstructive
Surgery, Assistant Professor, Department of
Otolaryngology–Head and Neck Surgery,
Harvard Medical School, Massachusetts Eye
and Ear, Associate Chief of Plastic Surgery,
Harvard Vanguard Medical Associates,
Boston, Massachusetts, USA

SAHAR NADIMI, MD
Department of Otolaryngology–Head and Neck
Surgery, Loyola University Medical Center,
Maywood, Illinois, USA; Chicago Hair Institute
(Private Practice), Oakbrook Terrace, Illinois,
USA

JELENA NIKOLIC, MD, PhD
Faculty of Medicine, University of Novi Sad,
Novi Sad, Serbia

JORDAN P. SAND, MD, FACS
Director, Spokane Center for Facial Plastic
Surgery, Spokane, Washington, USA

TYMON TAI, MD
Resident Physician, Tina and Rick Caruso
Department of Otolaryngology–Head and Neck
Surgery, Keck School of Medicine of USC, Los
Angeles, California, USA

SHANNON WATKINS, MD
Clinical Assistant Professor of Dermatology,
Weill Cornell Medical School, New York, New
York, USA

Contents

Androgenetic alopecia (AGA) is the most common hair loss disorder in men and women. The characteristic and reproducible balding pattern in AGA negatively affects self-image and the external perceptions of the balding patient. The phenotypical changes are driven by dihydrotestosterone (DHT) and its precursor testosterone. DHT induces follicle miniaturization and hair cycle changes until resulting hairs no longer extrude through the skin surface. AGA is inherited in a polygenetic pattern and is susceptible to epigenetic and environmental factors. Currently, minoxidil, finasteride, and photolaser therapy are the only Food and Drug Administration–approved medical treatments for AGA.

Hair transplant is a powerful and reliable procedure that provides a natural and high-impact result. This procedure can be used to restore scalp hair, eyebrow hair, beard hair, body hair, or areas of hair loss due to scarring. The hair transplant techniques of the past (hair plugs, scalp reductions) have etched a negative impression of hair restoration surgery in the public memory. With the improved techniques of follicular unit transplantation, more natural and discreet results can be obtained with minimal downtime and preservation of patient privacy. This article focuses on follicular unit transplantation and performance of the strip technique.

Hair transplantation, or hair restoration surgery (HRS) remains the only method to consistently restore hair in those experiencing pattern hair loss as well as hair loss from most other causes. HRS has been significantly improved with the development of follicular unit extraction, later renamed follicular unit excision, or FUE. This allows the surgeon to harvest grafts from the donor area without leaving a scar. FUE can also be used to harvest grafts from other areas of the body. When performed properly using the most technically advanced devices, the transection of the grafts with FUE remains under 4%.

Hair loss can be a debilitating condition, especially for individuals who already have chronic underlying medical conditions that complicate the treatment of hair loss.

This article addresses the challenges posed by scarring alopecia in hair-loss treatment and the evidence-based practices that exist for hair transplantation in scarring alopecia.

Platelet-rich plasma (PRP) is a promising treatment for hair restoration in patients with androgenic alopecia. Created from a platelet concentrate from an autologous blood draw, PRP is a safe therapeutic option for patients with hair loss. It is used alone or in conjunction with topical and oral therapies. Most studies of hair restoration with PRP report positive outcomes. Further research to optimize PRP preparation/administration procedures and identify patient populations that benefit most from this treatment are needed, as is long-term follow-up of objective hair loss outcomes. PRP appears to be a safe technology with excellent potential for promoting hair restoration.

Contemporary hair transplant surgery creates natural appearing transplanted hair. The procedure is performed as an outpatient under local anesthesia. Donor harvesting can be performed by either elliptical donor harvesting or follicular unit extraction. An experience surgical team is needed for a high-quality, efficient procedure. Robotic hair transplantation allows precise and efficient removal of follicular units. The robot allows for minimally invasive surgery. Robotic hair transplantation is an important tool for hair transplant surgeons, but does not replace appropriate candidate selection, hairline design, and the judgment of where to place and not place transplanted hair for optimal short- and long-term results.

As an alternative to hair transplantation for lowering the overly high hairline, hairline-lowering/forehead-reduction surgery has several advantages, including unsurpassed density and immediate results. Appropriate candidates for this surgery must have a stable frontal hairline (thus excluding most men) and a fairly to very mobile scalp that will permit sufficient advancement to warrant this more "invasive" approach. The main objective of this surgery is the lowering of the hairline. The authors' surgical approach, which was developed over the performance of more than 90 of these procedures and produces consistent results with low rates of complications, is described.

Hair restoration in women involves mastering both the medical and the surgical treatment. Preoperatively, women should be thoroughly evaluated for biochemical causes of hair loss along with a complete history and physical examination taken. The physician must recognize the clinical presentation of scarring alopecias and maintain a low threshold for biopsy to rule out this condition. Postoperative hair shock loss is a common feature following hair transplant in women, and the surgeon should understand the preoperative counseling and preventative measures needed, the intraoperative methods to reduce the incidence, and the postoperative strategies to handle the situation.

Sahar Nadimi

Most complications associated with hair transplant surgery are usually preventable and most often arise as a consequence of poor planning or faulty surgical technique. Patients should be evaluated for having realistic goals and a pattern that is amenable to aesthetic restoration. A good treatment plan must consider the potential for future hair loss. Well-informed patients who carefully follow instructions and take an active role in the postoperative recovery process minimize the chance of patient-controlled complications. This article discusses potential complications associated with hair restoration surgery, and the roles of the patient and physician in decreasing the risk of complications.

Anthony Bared

In the field of hair restoration, there has been a significant increase in demand with patients for facial hair transplantation procedures. Modern techniques in hair transplantation allow for facial hair transplantation and for the attainment of natural-appearing results. Facial hair transplantation is a subspecialty within hair restoration with many gratifying benefits for the patients as well as for the hair restoration surgeon. Adapting these advanced techniques into a hair restoration practice allows a surgeon to offer their patients these procedures and provides an expanded artistic element to a hair restoration surgeon's practice.

FACIAL PLASTIC SURGERY CLINICS OF NORTH AMERICA

SERIES OF RELATED INTEREST

Clinics in Plastic Surgery
https://www.plasticsurgery.theclinics.com
Otolaryngologic Clinics
https://www.oto.theclinics.com
Dermatologic Clinics
https://www.derm.theclinics.com

THE CLINICS ARE AVAILABLE ONLINE!
Access your subscription at:
www.theclinics.com

Foreword
Techniques for Hair Restoration

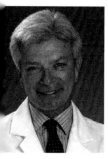

Regan Thomas, MD
Consulting Editor

Hair transplantation and related treatment modalities have greatly increased in interest and popularity in recent years. It has been noted that hair restoration has significant self-image and social interaction benefits to the patient population, and individuals are increasingly seeking appropriate treatment opportunities. A wide array of treatment options has been developed and can be of benefit to both genders who desire improvement and restoration of their hair loss. This issue of *Facial Plastic Surgery Clinics of North America* provides insight and review of a wide array of hair restoration technologies, procedures, and treatments that may be utilized to the benefit of the large patient population interested in hair restoration.

Drs Ishii and Lee as guest editors have explored the multiple treatment options and technologies available to these patient populations through the examples and descriptions of the expertise and experience of a number of selected expert contributing authors. The articles from these experts in the specialties of Dermatology and Facial Plastic Surgery include a wide range of treatments available, such as hair transplant surgeries, hair-lowering procedures, laser treatments, platelet-rich plasma injections, and medical therapies. In addition to discussing the multiple treatment options, Drs Ishii and Lee have selected authors who have documented experience and insights to providing the ideal treatment program for the individual patients desiring these treatment outcomes.

Hair restoration treatments and approaches have been rapidly growing, and new treatment options have been developed in the recent past. The selected group of contributing authors provides a thorough update of these treatments as well as outlines specific steps and considerations based on the patient's need. The expertise, descriptions, and experience in this issue will provide a valuable addition to the Facial Plastic Surgery literature in this aspect of the specialty.

J. Regan Thomas, MD
Facial Plastic and Reconstructive Surgery
Department of Otolaryngology–Head
and Neck Surgery
Northwestern University of Medicine
675 North Saint Clair Street
Suite 15-200
Chicago, IL 60611, USA

E-mail address:
Regan.Thomas@nm.org

Facial Plast Surg Clin N Am 28 (2020) ix
https://doi.org/10.1016/j.fsc.2020.02.002
1064-7406/20/© 2020 Published by Elsevier Inc.

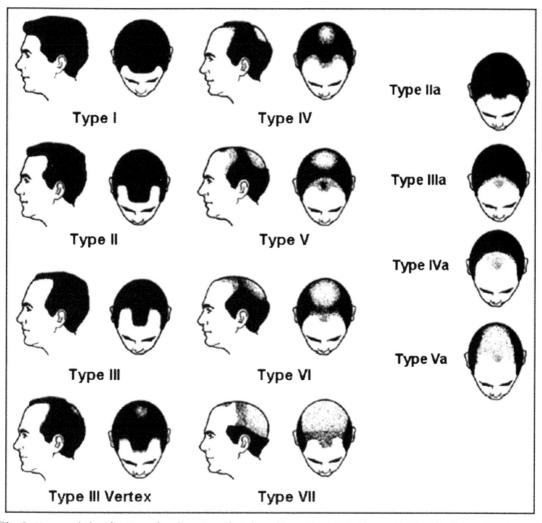

Fig. 2. Norwood classification of male pattern hair loss. (*From* Gupta M, Mysore V. Classifications of patterned hair loss: a review. J Cutan Aesthet Surg. 2016;9(1):3–12; with permission.)

binding, whereas hair follicles in the frontal scalp and vertex miniaturize as observed in MPHL.[12] The largely androgen-insensitive hair follicles in the occipital and temporal scalp are unaffected.

Embryologically, the frontoparietal scalp dermis arises from neural crest cells and the occipital and temporal scalp stem from mesodermal origins.[8] It is surmised that the differences in derivation lead to site-specific differences in hair growth. The success of modern hair transplant techniques relies on these differences; the donor dominance theory relies on hair follicles from the temporal and occipital region maintaining their androgen-independence even after they are relocated to areas of hair loss.

Testosterone is the primary systemically circulating androgen. It may directly bind to androgen receptors (AR) in the DPCs and hair bulb or it

can be converted to dihydrotestosterone (DHT) by 5-alpha reductase, allowing for a 5-fold increase in binding affinity to the AR compared with testosterone (**Fig. 3**). DHT is considered to be the dominant androgen responsible for inducing the hair follicle alterations seen in MPHL.[13] Two types of 5-alpha reductase mediate this conversion: type I 5-alpha reductase, which is found in the liver and brain, and type II, which is concentrated in the prostate, epididymis, and the DPCs affected in MPHL.[14]

Androgen receptor binding produces a downstream cascade of intracellular signaling via the Wnt/β-catenin pathway.[15–18] Molecular signaling also occurs via TGF-B1, a growth factor known to induce catagen, and TGF-β2, dickkpof1, and interleukin 6, established mediators of apoptosis and growth inhibition.[19–21] A positive feedback

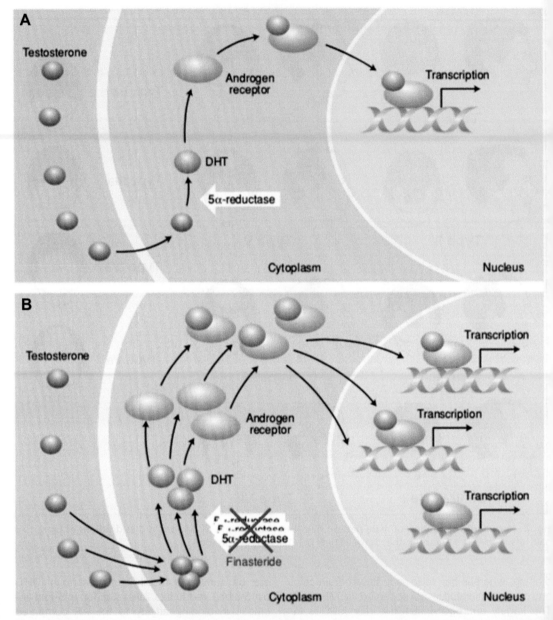

Fig. 3. Involvement of androgens and the androgen receptor in male pattern baldness. (*From* Ellis JA, Sinclair R, Harrap SB. Androgenetic alopecia: pathogenesis and potential for therapy. Expert Rev Mol Med. 2002;4(220):5; with permission.)

loop perpetuates when these factors are released, resulting in increased AR production and increased 5-alpha reductase levels. Other suspected mediators of hair follicle development have been seen in animal model experiments.[12,22,23]

Alternative non–androgen-dependent pathways are suspected in the pathophysiology of FPHL. Early studies of MPHL in hypogonadal men by Hamilton[9] demonstrated that castration before puberty effectively prevented MPHL, whereas subsequent testosterone injections in these men could induce baldness. In contrast, AGA has been documented in women with androgen insensitivity syndrome, implying that FPHL operates via androgen-independent mechanisms.[24]

Lower levels of 5-alpha reductase and the presence of cytochrome P450 aromatase in women, which competitively converts testosterone into estradriol and estrone at the xpense of DHT, create a different hormonal milieu in the female scalp. The higher aromatase evels found in the frontal and occipital regions f the female scalp are suspected to confer a rotective effect against hair loss in these egions.[25]

nvironmental Factors

Oxidative stress is also a factor involved in MPHL. tudies subjecting in vitro cultured DPCs to varying levels of O2 saturations demonstrate ecreased growth and higher levels of reactive oxygen species in atmospheric O2 than when subjected to physiologic O2 levels.[26] Balding scalp DPCs grow slower than DPCs from occipital scalp n response to these environmental changes.

Genetic Factors

MPHL exhibits a polygenic inheritance pattern with associated gene loci located in both sexnked and autosomal chromosomes. The first discovered heritable element in MPHL is a single-nucleotide polymorphism (SNP) in exon1 f the androgen receptor gene on chromosome . Genome-wide association studies demonstrate hat this SNP is nearly ubiquitous in patients with MPHL and is also present in large proportions of older nonbalding men, suggesting that this SNP s required but is not solely responsible for the manifestation of MPHL.[27]

Similarly, the incidence of a Stu1 gene polymorphism is linked with male baldness. A greater Stu1 SNP length is associated with increased AR xpression and increased risk for MPHL.[28]

GWAS studies have also identified several other uspect loci: genes on chromosomes 3q26, p21.1, and 20p11 are strongly linked with MPHL, but their androgen-independent pathways or inducing baldness remains unclear.[29–32] In hort, numerous genetic loci are known to permit r inhibit MPHL, but specific therapeutic targets ave yet to be determined.

Genetic studies into female balding have yet to ssociate FHPL incidence with specific genomic lements. Experiments aiming to link FPHL with he female sex steroid pathway, aromatase genes, r estrogen receptor genes have proved unsuccessful. There have not been any demonstrable ssociations between FPHL and the previously mentioned susceptibility loci identified in MPHL.[33]

pigenetic Factors

he dermal papillae cells of nonbalding follicles ave been shown to be less rich in androgen receptors than those of balding follicles.[34] Across he scalp, epigenetic alterations in the androgen

receptor pathway further propagate activating or inhibitory effects on site-specific hair follicle growth. For one, DNA methylation of the AR gene promoter sequence, which results in decreased AR expression, is a more prevalent epigenetic pattern in the occipital scalp hair follicles than in the vertex of patients with MPHL. This provides one more explanation for the preservation of occipital hair in MPHL. Promoter hypomethylation of the AR promoter has the opposite effect, upregulating AR expression.[35] The exclusive presence of molecular coactivators such as Hic-5/ARA55 in the DPCs in the androgen-dependent frontoparietal and vertex regions has also been shown to contribute to androgen sensitivity.[36] These observed changes contributing to hair loss persist in the epigenetic profiles of affected offspring.

MEDICAL THERAPY

As of publication, minoxidil, finasteride, and low-level laser light therapy (LLLT) are the 3 Food and Drug Administration (FDA)-approved modalities for nonsurgical treatment of MPHL. The highest levels of evidence support the efficacy of minoxidil and finasteride in balding patients; however, both medications require continual use to maintain their desired effects. LLLT is a useful alternative for patients who do not tolerate minoxidil or finasteride due to side effects or have difficulty with administration. Several other pharmaceutical agents including dutasteride are prescribed for the off-label treatment of MPHL and FPHL. These drugs are discussed in the following section. The use of supplements and nonprescription alternatives are frequently areas of patient interest; their efficacy and safety profiles are also reviewed.

Minoxidil

Originally advertised as an antihypertensive agent, minoxidil became approved for the first-line treatment of AGA after the realization of its hypertrichosis effects. It is available as a 2% and 5% topical solution, requires twice daily topical application, and needs to be maintained for at least 4 hours on the scalp for each application. On skin contact, minoxidil is converted to minoxidil sulfate, which potentiates potassium channels in smooth muscle. The smooth muscle relaxes, hair follicle perfusion increases, and the anagen phase extends, delaying conversion from terminal to vellus hair.[37]

Effects in men

Multiple double-blinded randomized control studies have established the efficacy of minoxidil in increasing hair weight and diameter.[38] Aesthetic results are appreciable after 16 weeks of use and should be assessed by the physician at 6 months. There is no evidence to suggest that minoxidil's effects stem from reversing previously miniaturized hair follicles but rather from slowing disease progression and preventing further miniaturization. The 5% formulation is shown to produce slightly improved cosmetic results (60%) compared with that of the 2% formulation (40%).[39] Patients should be cautioned about a temporary telogen effluvium within the first month of minoxidil use. The patient should continue the treatment, as this shedding is self-limited and is seen before the hair growth period. The patient should also understand that minoxidil requires routine application to maintain its effects, otherwise MPHL will recur.

The most cited adverse effects of minoxidil include contact dermatitis, tachycardia, and hypertrichosis. Skin irritation is remedied by switching to the lower dose 2% formulation or a propylene glycol-free foam preparation. Care should be taken to avoid leaving residual medication on pillows and bedsheets that can come into contact with the face; application several hours before bed decreases this risk. Hypertrichosis from accidental application to nonscalp skin reverses approximately 1 month after the drug is discontinued. Patients with cardiovascular disease are advised to avoid minoxidil because tachycardia has been reported, although no resulting adverse effects have been documented.

Effects in women

For women, minoxidil is sold as a 2% formulation. Blume-Peytavi and colleagues[38] demonstrated equal efficacy with twice daily application of the 2% lotion compared with a daily application of the 5% foam. The most frequent complication from minoxidil use in women is hypertrichosis. Again, hypertrichosis resolves 1 to 3 months after discontinuation. Pregnant women should avoid minoxidil as its teratogenic profile is not well established in human studies.

Finasteride

By selectively inhibiting 5-alpha reductase type 2 production of DHT, a once-daily 5-mg tablet of finasteride produces the most effective results among the 3 modalities approved by the FDA for MPHL.[40,41] Improvements are observed mainly in hair width and growth rate, as the truncated anagen phase is restored to its previous length.[42] Improvements in scalp appearance are observable as early as 12 weeks; formal evaluation should be performed after 6 months of use.

For women, finasteride is not FDA approved for the treatment of FPHL. Yeon and colleagues[43] demonstrated improvements in hair density, width, and scalp appearance after 1 year of finasteride use for a small population of Asian women. Another study purported subjective improvements combining finasteride and oral contraceptives compared with placebo.[44] Overall, although data validating improvements in hair width and growth rate with finasteride use in the female population are inconsistent and its use is not recommended.

The most common side effects from finasteride use in MPHL are decreased libido, erectile dysfunction, and gynecomastia. Depression has also been reported after finasteride use. Nusbaum and colleagues[45] submitted previously in this journal that their patients experienced resolution of these side effects after switching from a daily to every other day dosing schedule. Permanent sexual side effects in men have been described but are poorly substantiated in large randomized control trials. Most of the patients experience resolution of these side effects after discontinuing the drug.

Men who undergo prostate-specific androgen (PSA) monitoring for prostate cancer should be counseled that finasteride reduces serum PSA levels. Physicians should be aware of this medication when obtaining the patient's history and compensate by doubling the measured serum level when evaluating PSA. There is a growing body of evidence suggesting that finasteride use is not linked with an increased risk of prostate cancer nor does it induce lower sperm count.[46,47]

Because of its antiandrogenic effects, pregnant women are advised against coming into physical contact with finasteride. Doing so may inhibit the proper sexual development of male fetuses or induce genital abnormalities. However, finasteride does not affect sperm and can be safely used by sexually active men without risk to a developing fetus.

Combination Therapy

Combining minoxidil lotion with oral finasteride tablets improves the appearance of the balding scalp as described by the patient and to clinical evaluators compared with either therapy alone. This same study describes the use of finasteride in conjunction with ketoconazole or as monotherapy to be more effective than minoxidil only.[4] Minoxidil or finasteride before hair transplantation may also mitigate the postoperative shedding phase that frequently develops.[48] The amount of transplanted hair lost is reduced with adjunctive medical therapy and should be considered during the surgical consultation.

Dutasteride

Dutasteride nonselectively inhibits types I and II 5-alpha reductase. This higher-affinity finasteride analogue is FDA approved for benign prostatic hyperplasia but is used off-label for its follicle-stimulating effects. Patients taking oral dutasteride experience increased hair density and improved subjective appearance on photographic assessment of the scalp.[49]

A 2.5-mg daily dose of dutasteride yields more hair growth than the standard 5-mg daily dose of finasteride. However, the increased potency of dutasteride translates to a higher incidence of finasteride-like side effects, including loss of libido, erectile dysfunction, and gynecomastia.[50] Physicians prescribing dutasteride for off-label use should include these risks when providing guidance to patients. Because of its established efficacy and safety profile, dutasteride can be considered if patients are refractory to first-line treatment.

Photolaser Therapy

In LLLT, photons from laser light are hypothesized to stimulate the mitochondrial cytochrome oxidase system. Production of O_2 and ATP increases and follicular apoptosis is abated. Hair growth can be witnessed as early after 4 weeks of use. The laser is emitted from a handheld device akin to a hairbrush or as a cap that covers the entire scalp. In-home and in-office systems demonstrate comparable efficacy in stimulating hair growth. Both options require three 10- to 15-minute sessions per week. This frequent treatment schedule may be prohibitive for some patients. The European Academy of Dermatology and Venereology guidelines report photolaser therapy as a safe and effective adjunct therapy for AGA in men and women, although long-term efficacy data are insufficient.[38] A separate systematic review by Delaney and Zhang[51] reaches similar conclusions that LLLT is generally safe and well tolerated. Patients may note short-term scalp itching, dryness, and tenderness from use.

Hormone Treatments

Antiandrogenic agents including spironolactone, cyproterone acetate, and fluridil, a topical androgen receptor binder, are used as off-label medications for pattern hair loss. Individualized trials have demonstrated hair regrowth in women using spironolactone, cyproterone, or fluridil.[52,53] In the same systematic review performed by the European Academy of Dermatology and Venereology, neither oral or topical antiandrogens could be recommended in the treatment of hair loss except for cyproterone acetate in hyperandrogenic women.[38]

Prostaglandins

Topical bimatoprost, a prostaglandin D2 analogue, is indicated for enhancing eyelash and eyebrow hair. As mentioned previously, the prostaglandin D2 (PGD_2) pathway is inhibitory to hair growth. Activation of this inhibitory pathway occurs at higher concentrations in the balding scalp than in other hair-bearing regions.[22] These associations propose bimatoprost as a potential third pharmaceutical agent in AGA treatment, but as of this journal's earlier review of nonsurgical hair loss therapies in 2013 robust clinical trials have yet to be published. A small randomized double-blind study (n = 16) demonstrated increased hair density after 24 weeks of treatment with 0.1% latanoprost, a $PGF_{2\alpha}$ analogue commonly marketed for eyelash lengthening.[54–57] Further validation studies are needed.

Supplementation

The production and marketing of vitamins and supplements remains loosely regulated: hair loss products that claim to restore hair length and density are poorly substantiated by experimental data. Saw palmetto (Serenoa repens) is a plant extract used in benign prostatic hyperplasia for its 5-alpha reductase inhibition in the prostate gland. A single randomized, double-blind controlled study demonstrated increased hair growth in 6 of 10 patients with MPHL with saw palmetto use.[58] Otherwise, no clinical trials have been performed evaluating the efficacy of biotin, nioxin, procerin, or topical serums. Niacin, amino acids, vitamins, hibiscus, red ginseng, melatonin, and botulinum toxin are other compounds also not routinely recommended due to limited experimental data.[38] Patients should be informed of the low levels of evidence surrounding these products in the interest of making informed treatment decisions.

Cosmetic Aids

Hairpieces with synthetic or natural hair fibers are appropriate alternatives if patients do not desire or are unable to tolerate other treatments. These aids offer the appearance of natural hair with a high level of fidelity. Sprays and powders darken hair and camouflage the scalp, creating the appearance of thicker hair. Patients unsatisfied with the results of medical or surgical therapy can consider this as a helpful adjunct.

Considerations for the Transgender Patient

Trans women, phenotypic men who identify with the female gender, and trans men, phenotypic women who identify with the male gender, often undergo hormone therapy to induce the development of secondary sex characteristics of their chosen identity. The aim of feminization hormone therapy is to stimulate breast tissue and adipose tissue growth in addition to augmenting the growth of facial hair and body hair in a typical female distribution. This can be achieved primarily with estrogen therapy, although nonestrogen hormones such as leuprolide, spironolactone, and flutamide are viable substitutes.[59] For trans men, testosterone administration suppresses female secondary sex characteristics and stimulates hair growth in a characteristically male pattern that involves the face and chest.[60]

Oral or transdermal estrogen therapy for the trans woman impedes hair growth in the body and face. Follicle size, density, and growth rate decrease over the treatment course of 18 to 24 months. The resulting appearance is thinner, less-dense hair and the absence of hair along the cheek, jaw, and chin.

Trans women who are at risk for or experiencing MPHL can elect to use finasteride or minoxidil to treat hair loss with a high degree of success.[61] The estrogen from feminization therapy poses no reported risk of FPHL induction and in fact has been shown to counteract the physiologic changes of MPHL. The addition of antiandrogens such as spironolactone can also be considered for its testosterone-lowering effect. A combination of estrogen, minoxidil, and spironolactone can be used safely for trans women affected by MPHL without the risk of developing MPHL.[62]

Testosterone therapy for trans men produces thicker, denser facial and body hair alongside increased acne, sebum, muscle mass, libido, a deepening voice, and clitoromegaly noticeable after 12 weeks of treatment. Over time, these hormonal changes induce hair cycle changes and follicular miniaturization in the frontotemporal distribution described in MPHL. The incidence of MPHL in trans men undergoing testosterone therapy ranges from 17% to 33%.[63,64] It is important to discuss these changes with the patient and whether they are desired or not—certain patients may consider this male-pattern hair loss as feature that enhances their masculine characteristics, whereas others may find the appearance unappealing.

If the female-to-male patient desires treatment of their AGA, topical minoxidil is the treatment of choice. No adverse effects with testosterone therapy have been reported. Finasteride for the trans man should be carefully considered before administration. Although oral finasteride in trans men has been shown to be effective in the treatment of MPHL, studies on its sexual side effects in this population lack statistical power. In addition, the inhibitory effects of finasteride may prevent potentially desired secondary sex characteristics such as voice deepening, body hair, and body habitus changes from taking place.[65] Another important consideration is the patient's desire for fertility. Patients who have not undergone oophorectomy with hysterectomy are fertile after the cessation of testosterone therapy. Therefore, finasteride use is strictly prohibited in trans men who have the potential for pregnancy due to concern for inducing fetal developmental abnormalities.[66]

SUMMARY

The basic mechanisms for AGA are now well understood to arise from the interactions of testosterone and DHT on scalp androgen receptors. Advances in molecular biology and genetic analysis techniques have been brought to bear, providing deeper understanding of the phenotypic variation of AGA along the scalp and identifying potential targets for future genetic or drug therapies. To date, no new interventions are used routinely in the treatment of AGA. Minoxidil and finasteride remain the mainstays of medical therapy with well-established safety and efficacy profiles as long as they are continually administered. Along with low-light laser therapy, these agents are approved by the FDA for treatment of AGA. Other agents such as antiandrogens are used on an off-label basis and should be carefully reviewed with the patient before its use. Finally, transgender men and women are a unique population of hair loss patients that require a nuanced discussion of treatment considerations and expectations. The role on the clinician in establishing these expectations is paramount both in cis and transgender populations.

DISCLOSURE

The authors have nothing to disclose.

REFERENCES

1. Cash TF. The psychological effects of androgenetic alopecia in men. J Am Acad Dermatol 1992;26(6):926–31.
2. Cash TF, Price VH, Savin RC. Psychological effects of androgenetic alopecia on women: comparisons

with balding men and with female control subjects. J Am Acad Dermatol 1993;29(4):568–75.

3. Ellis JA, Sinclair R, Harrap SB. Androgenetic alopecia: pathogenesis and potential for therapy. Expert Rev Mol Med 2002;4(22):1–11.

4. Severi G, Sinclair R, Hopper JL, et al. Androgenetic alopecia in men aged 40-69 years: prevalence and risk factors. Br J Dermatol 2003;149(6):1207–13.

5. Paik JH, Yoon JB, Sim WY, et al. The prevalence and types of androgenetic alopecia in Korean men and women. Br J Dermatol 2001;145(1):95–9.

6. Martel JL, Badri T. Anatomy, hair follicle. Treasure Island (FL): StatPearls; 2019.

7. Paus R, Cotsarelis G. The biology of hair follicles. N Engl J Med 1999;341(7):491–7.

8. Banka N, Bunagan MJ, Shapiro J. Pattern hair loss in men: diagnosis and medical treatment. Dermatol Clin 2013;31(1):129–40.

9. Hamilton JB. Patterned loss of hair in man; types and incidence. Ann N Y Acad Sci 1951;53(3): 708–28.

10. Norwood OT. Male pattern baldness: classification and incidence. South Med J 1975;68(11): 1359–65.

11. Ludwig E. Classification of the types of androgenetic alopecia (common baldness) occurring in the female sex. Br J Dermatol 1977;97(3):247–54.

12. Lolli F, Pallotti F, Rossi A, et al. Androgenetic alopecia: a review. Endocrine 2017;57(1):9–17.

13. Kaufman KD. Androgens and alopecia. Mol Cell Endocrinol 2002;198(1–2):89–95.

14. Russell DW, Berman DM, Bryant JT, et al. The molecular genetics of steroid 5 alpha-reductases. Recent Prog Horm Res 1994;49:275–84.

15. Chesire DR, Isaacs WB. Ligand-dependent inhibition of beta-catenin/TCF signaling by androgen receptor. Oncogene 2002;21(55):8453–69.

16. Leiros GJ, Attorresi AI, Balana ME. Hair follicle stem cell differentiation is inhibited through cross-talk between Wnt/beta-catenin and androgen signalling in dermal papilla cells from patients with androgenetic alopecia. Br J Dermatol 2012;166(5):1035–42.

17. Li R, Brockschmidt FF, Kiefer AK, et al. Six novel susceptibility Loci for early-onset androgenetic alopecia and their unexpected association with common diseases. PLoS Genet 2012;8(5):e1002746.

18. Rodlor E, Dobson K, Drichel D, et al. Investigation of six novel susceptibility loci for male androgenetic alopecia in women with female pattern hair loss. J Dermatol Sci 2013;72(2):186–8.

19. Inui S, Itami S. Molecular basis of androgenetic alopecia: from androgen to paracrine mediators through dermal papilla. J Dermatol Sci 2011;61(1): 1–6.

20. Kwack MH, Ahn JS, Kim MK, et al. Dihydrotestosterone-inducible IL-6 inhibits elongation of human hair shafts by suppressing matrix cell proliferation and promotes regression of hair follicles in mice. J Invest Dermatol 2012;132(1):43–9.

21. Hibino T, Nishiyama T. Role of TGF-beta2 in the human hair cycle. J Dermatol Sci 2004;35(1):9–18.

22. Garza LA, Liu Y, Yang Z, et al. Prostaglandin D2 inhibits hair growth and is elevated in bald scalp of men with androgenetic alopecia. Sci Transl Med 2012;4(126):126ra134.

23. Heilmann S, Nyholt DR, Brockschmidt FF, et al. No genetic support for a contribution of prostaglandins to the aetiology of androgenetic alopecia. Br J Dermatol 2013;169(1):222–4.

24. Cousen P, Messenger A. Female pattern hair loss in complete androgen insensitivity syndrome. Br J Dermatol 2010;162(5):1135–7.

25. Sawaya ME, Price VH. Different levels of 5alpha-reductase type I and II, aromatase, and androgen receptor in hair follicles of women and men with androgenetic alopecia. J Invest Dermatol 1997; 109(3):296–300.

26. Upton JH, Hannen RF, Bahta AW, et al. Oxidative stress-associated senescence in dermal papilla cells of men with androgenetic alopecia. J Invest Dermatol 2015;135(5):1244–52.

27. Ellis JA, Stebbing M, Harrap SB. Polymorphism of the androgen receptor gene is associated with male pattern baldness. J Invest Dermatol 2001; 116(3):452–5.

28. Ellis JA, Scurrah KJ, Cobb JE, et al. Baldness and the androgen receptor: the AR polyglycine repeat polymorphism does not confer susceptibility to androgenetic alopecia. Hum Genet 2007;121(3–4): 451–7.

29. Hillmer AM, Brockschmidt FF, Hanneken S, et al. Susceptibility variants for male-pattern baldness on chromosome 20p11. Nat Genet 2008;40(11): 1279–81.

30. Hillmer AM, Flaquer A, Hanneken S, et al. Genome-wide scan and fine-mapping linkage study of androgenetic alopecia reveals a locus on chromosome 3q26. Am J Hum Genet 2008;82(3):737–43.

31. Brockschmidt FF, Heilmann S, Ellis JA, et al. Susceptibility variants on chromosome 7p21.1 suggest HDAC9 as a new candidate gene for male-pattern baldness. Br J Dermatol 2011;165(6):1293–302.

32. Richards JB, Yuan X, Geller F, et al. Male-pattern baldness susceptibility locus at 20p11. Nat Genet 2008;40(11):1282–4.

33. Redler S, Messenger AG, Betz RC. Genetics and other factors in the aetiology of female pattern hair loss. Exp Dermatol 2017;26(6):510–7.

34. Hibberts NA, Howell AE, Randall VA. Balding hair follicle dermal papilla cells contain higher levels of androgen receptors than those from non-balding scalp. J Endocrinol 1998;156(1):59–65.

35. Cobb JE, Wong NC, Yip LW, et al. Evidence of increased DNA methylation of the androgen receptor

gene in occipital hair follicles from men with androgenetic alopecia. Br J Dermatol 2011;165(1):210–3.

36. Randall VA, Thornton MJ, Messenger AG. Cultured
dermal papilla cells from androgen-dependent human hair follicles (e.g. beard) contain more
androgen receptors than those from non-balding
areas of scalp. J Endocrinol 1992;133(1):141–7.

37. Li M, Marubayashi A, Nakaya Y, et al. Minoxidil-
induced hair growth is mediated by adenosine in
cultured dermal papilla cells: possible involvement
of sulfonylurea receptor 2B as a target of minoxidil.
J Invest Dermatol 2001;117(6):1594–600.

38. Kanti V, Messenger A, Dobos G, et al. Evidence-
based (S3) guideline for the treatment of androgenetic alopecia in women and in men - short
version. J Eur Acad Dermatol Venereol 2018;
32(1):11–22.

39. Olsen EA, Dunlap FE, Funicella T, et al.
A randomized clinical trial of 5% topical minoxidil
versus 2% topical minoxidil and placebo in the treatment of androgenetic alopecia in men. J Am Acad
Dermatol 2002;47(3):377–85.

40. Khandpur S, Suman M, Reddy BS. Comparative efficacy of various treatment regimens for androgenetic alopecia in men. J Dermatol 2002;29(8):
489–98.

41. Adil A, Godwin M. The effectiveness of treatments
for androgenetic alopecia: a systematic review and
meta-analysis. J Am Acad Dermatol 2017;77(1):
136–41.e5.

42. Whiting DA, Waldstreicher J, Sanchez M, et al.
Measuring reversal of hair miniaturization in androgenetic alopecia by follicular counts in horizontal
sections of serial scalp biopsies: results of finasteride 1 mg treatment of men and postmenopausal
women. J Investig Dermatol Symp Proc 1999;4(3):
282–4.

43. Yeon JH, Jung JY, Choi JW, et al. 5 mg/day finasteride treatment for normoandrogenic Asian women
with female pattern hair loss. J Eur Acad Dermatol
Venereol 2011;25(2):211–4.

44. Iorizzo M, Vincenzi C, Voudouris S, et al. Finasteride
treatment of female pattern hair loss. Arch Dermatol
2006;142(3):298–302.

45. Nusbaum AG, Rose PT, Nusbaum BP. Nonsurgical
therapy for hair loss. Facial Plast Surg Clin North
Am 2013;21(3):335–42.

46. Andriole GL, Humphrey PA, Serfling RJ, et al. High-
grade prostate cancer in the Prostate Cancer Prevention Trial: fact or artifact? J Natl Cancer Inst
2007;99(18):1355–6.

47. Rogers NE, Avram MR. Medical treatments for male
and female pattern hair loss. J Am Acad Dermatol
2008;59(4):547–66 [quiz: 567–8].

48. Kassimir JJ. Use of topical minoxidil as a possible
adjunct to hair transplant surgery. A pilot study.
J Am Acad Dermatol 1987;16(3 Pt 2):685–7.

49. Stough D. Dutasteride improves male pattern hair
loss in a randomized study in identical twins.
J Cosmet Dermatol 2007;6(1):9–13.

50. Olsen EA, Hordinsky M, Whiting D, et al. The importance of dual 5alpha-reductase inhibition in the
treatment of male pattern hair loss: results of a randomized placebo-controlled study of dutasteride
versus finasteride. J Am Acad Dermatol 2006;
55(6):1014–23.

51. Delaney SW, Zhang P. Systematic review of low-level
laser therapy for adult androgenic alopecia.
J Cosmet Laser Ther 2018;20(4):229–36.

52. Sinclair R, Wewerinke M, Jolley D. Treatment of female pattern hair loss with oral antiandrogens. Br J
Dermatol 2005;152(3):466–73.

53. Vexiau P, Chaspoux C, Boudou P, et al. Effects of
minoxidil 2% vs. cyproterone acetate treatment on
female androgenetic alopecia: a controlled, 12-
month randomized trial. Br J Dermatol 2002;146(6):
992–9.

54. Blume-Peytavi U, Lonnfors S, Hillmann K, et al.
A randomized double-blind placebo-controlled pilot
study to assess the efficacy of a 24-week topical
treatment by latanoprost 0.1% on hair growth and
pigmentation in healthy volunteers with androgenetic alopecia. J Am Acad Dermatol 2012;66(5):
794–800.

55. Gkini MA, Kouskoukis AE, Tripsianis G, et al. Study
of platelet-rich plasma injections in the treatment of
androgenetic alopecia through an one-year period.
J Cutan Aesthet Surg 2014;7(4):213–9.

56. Schiavone G, Raskovic D, Greco J, et al. Platelet-
rich plasma for androgenetic alopecia: a pilot study.
Dermatol Surg 2014;40(9):1010–9.

57. Sand JP, Nabili V, Kochhar A, et al. Platelet-rich
plasma for the aesthetic surgeon. Facial Plast Surg
2017;33(4):437–43.

58. Prager N, Bickett K, French N, et al. A randomized
double-blind, placebo-controlled trial to determine
the effectiveness of botanically derived inhibitors of
5-alpha-reductase in the treatment of androgenetic
alopecia. J Altern Complement Med 2002;8(2):
143–52.

59. Giltay EJ, Gooren LJ. Effects of sex steroid depriva-
tion/administration on hair growth and skin sebum
production in transsexual males and females.
J Clin Endocrinol Metab 2000;85(8):2913–21.

60. Irwig MS. Testosterone therapy for transgender men.
Lancet Diabetes Endocrinol 2017;5(4):301–11.

61. Stevenson MO, Wixon N, Safer JD. Scalp hair regrowth in hormone-treated transgender woman.
Transgend Health 2016;1(1):202–4.

62. Gao Y, Maurer T, Mirmirani P. Understanding and ad-
dressing hair disorders in transgender individuals.
Am J Clin Dermatol 2018;19(4):517–27.

63. Wierckx K, Van Caenegem E, Schreiner T, et al.
Cross-sex hormone therapy in trans persons is

safe and effective at short-time follow-up: results from the European network for the investigation of gender incongruence. J Sex Med 2014;11(8): 1999–2011.

64. Wierckx K, Van de Peer F, Verhaeghe E, et al. Short- and long-term clinical skin effects of testosterone treatment in trans men. J Sex Med 2014;11(1): 222–9.

65. Ginsberg BA. Dermatologic care of the transgender patient. Int J Womens Dermatol 2017;3(1):65–7.

66. Rittmaster RS. Finasteride. N Engl J Med 1994; 330(2):120–5.

Follicular Unit Transplantation

Jordan P. Sand, MD, FACS

KEYWORDS

• Hair transplantation • Follicular unit • Hair restoration

KEY POINTS

- Follicular unit transplantation (FUT) involves removing occipital scalp tissue, microscopically dissecting the follicular units, and then reimplanting them into areas of concern.
- FUT is a highly reliable procedure, with expected graft survival greater than 95% when using proper techniques.
- FUT does leave an occipital scar, but with trichophytic incisions, the scar is low impact.

INTRODUCTION

Hair transplant is a powerful and reliable procedure that provides a natural and high-impact result. This procedure can be used to restore scalp hair, eyebrow hair, beard hair, body hair, or areas of hair loss due to scarring. The hair transplant techniques of the past (hair plugs) have etched a negative impression of hair restoration surgery in the public memory. With the improved techniques of follicular unit transplantation, more natural and discreet results can be obtained with minimal downtime and preservation of patient privacy. These updated techniques leave less of a stigma associated with historical hair transplants along with improved results. This article focuses on follicular unit transplantation and performance of the strip technique.

HAIR TRANSPLANTATION

For the male or female patient suffering from hair loss, the personal and social impact from signs of aging has been a long-standing concern, which is well reflected in the multitude of age-old tonics and treatments that have been marketed. In the practice of facial plastic surgery, male patients will often present with concerns regarding their hair thinning and loss. In society, a full and lush head of hair is associated with youth and vitality. In addition, when the frontal hairline is restored,

facial balance is improved. Although these can be addressed with cosmetic treatments, male patients are particularly sensitive to both downtime and an unnatural surgical look. The holy grail of cosmetic surgery is to be able to perform a procedure in which the result is natural and difficult to detect as surgical and is associated with minimal recovery. Hair restoration follows this algorithm as a powerful tool to improve both the male and the female hairline with a high-impact outcome, little downtime, and a low risk of adverse events.

Hair restoration has evolved tremendously in recent history. Some of the initial reports around hair restoration are identified from Japan in 1939 by a physician who used full-thickness autografts to help perform facial hair restoration.[1] Further research has led to 2 key concepts for hair transplant that underpin the current surgical model: donor dominance and the follicular unit. The first concept of donor dominance describes the idea that transplanted autografts maintain their original growth characteristics. This autograft hypothesis was described by Orentreich,[2] who demonstrated the growth of occipital and parietal hair grafts placed into the frontal scalps of men with thinning hair. Interestingly, these grafts retained the original characteristics reflected from their donor site rather than taking on the features of the recipient site. Thus, they were not subject to the hormonally related loss of male-pattern baldness. Using this

Spokane Center for Facial Plastic Surgery, 217 West Cataldo Avenue, Third Floor, Spokane, WA 99201, USA
E-mail address: drsand@sandplasticsurgery.com

Facial Plast Surg Clin N Am 28 (2020) 161–167
https://doi.org/10.1016/j.fsc.2020.01.005
1064-7406/20/

finding, surgeons began treating patients with 4-mm punch grafts taken from the posterior scalp and transplanted to the frontal scalp. A session of hair restoration would involve taking about 100 of these "plug" grafts, each of which contained 20 to 30 hairs each. This type of hair restoration procedure was used for about 30 years, but left patients with a "pluggy" look and an unnatural-appearing hairline.[3]

THE FOLLICULAR UNIT

The second concept that is most responsible for the modern-day refinement of hair transplantation technique was the concept of the follicular unit. Elucidating the anatomic concepts of the follicular unit would permit for the development of micro-grafts and minigrafts to overcome the use of un-natural looking 4-mm punch grafts. In the early 1980s, micrografts of 3 to 6 hairs began to be described for use in the frontal hairline for a more natural appearance.[4] Further building on this finding, surgeons began using these micrografts on the entire scalp during a transplant session to further improve the cosmetic result.[5] Simultaneously, the follicular unit began to be better described in histologic studies. Studies by Headington[6] evaluated follicular units with horizontal sections and identified that "the follicular unit consisted of two to four terminal follicles, one or sometimes two vellus follicles, sebaceous lobules and also the insertions of the arrector pili muscle at the level of the mid dermis." A mean density of 100 FU/cm^2 was described in this with variation of 80 FU/cm^2 to 120 FU/cm^2.[6] However, later studies have considered that this was likely an overestimate of the follicular unit density.[7]

Further evaluation of the anatomy identified that 1 follicular unit may actually have between 1 and 5 terminal hair follicles, 1 or 2 vellus follicles, the associated sebaceous lobules, insertions of the arrector pili muscles, neural and vascular plexuses, and some fine adventitial collagen.[7,8] As an understanding of the microscopic anatomy built, the use of these follicles as the substrate for hair transplant began to gain traction. In the mid-1990s, surgeons began to describe the use of follicular unit transplantation, which quickly took over as the dominant method for hair transplant because of the superior aesthetic results it provides.[9–12]

PATIENT SELECTION

Although many patients can benefit from this procedure, the surgeon's selection process and planning are vital for a longer-term strategy to address a patient's hair loss, because this is a lifelong, progressive condition. By the age of 40, most men will identify a decline in their hair loss, but it is challenging to know what trajectory an even younger patient may take. The surgeon should complete a comprehensive history and examination because clues to the patient's genetic predisposition for hair loss can begin to be established. In addition, younger patients present early in the hair loss cycle and may have unrealistic expectations as to what hair restoration may provide. The sequelae of poor surgical planning include creating a too-low, unnatural hairline that is very challenging to correct as the native hairs continue to recede. Most hair restoration surgeons would not transplant a patient in their early to mid 20s for several reasons. First, the future cannot be accurately predicted with regard to any 1 individual's hair loss. With more time, hair loss patterns can be better diagnosed and prognosticated, so that the hair restoration surgeon can better avoid transplant in patients who will not have a long-term benefit. Thus, waste of the donor supply and creation of unnatural hairlines can be avoided. Second, the expectation of a younger patient is to maintain their youthful hairline, which is often unsustainable. For these younger patients, the default should be medical treatment to maintain their hair count and hair shaft size, also allowing time for the patient to mature their expectations of what can be provided with hair restoration.

EVALUATION OF DONOR AREA

A key step in creating a surgical plan for a patient is a thorough evaluation of the patient's donor area. This physical evaluation can help define the best course of action during the preoperative consultation and help make an informed decision about the surface to be treated with hair transplant. The donor area should be evaluated for the number of hairs per surface unit, the density of hairs per follicular unit, the color and texture of the hair and skin, the laxity and thickness of the scalp, and the texture of the hair. These qualities will help with planning the size and width of the strip and estimating the number of hairs available for transplant.

Currently, the follicular unit transplantation technique is the ideal method for restoration. Although advances in cloning and stem cell science have been made by researchers around the world, we do not yet have an unlimited supply of cloned hairs to use. Because of this, there are limitations to the number of hairs that can be transplanted. For most men, the occipital donor bank contains 6000 to 10,000 hairs that can be used.[3] Thus, an understanding of how to maximize the aesthetic distribution of these hairs is absolutely essential. On average, it is generally considered that the posterior scalp has 80 to 100 follicular units per squared centimeter. As each follicular unit will contain an average of 2.3 hairs, this works out to about 230 hairs per squared centimeter of scalp. Notably, significant hair loss can occur before it can be cosmetically identified. Once a patient's hair has thinned to approximately 50% of its native density, it begins to look thin. As a corollary, a transplanted density aiming for 50% of native density should provide excellent aesthetic scalp coverage.

Thus, when planning for hair transplantation, all of these factors should be considered by the surgeon. Again, because there is a limited donor supply, and because the patient is facing a progressive hair loss, there will always be an issue of supply and demand. The transplanted density also faces physical limitations because the follicles can only be placed so close together without compromising microvascular blood supply, and therefore, graft survival. Transplanting 25 follicular units per squared centimeter will provide a density just more than 50 hairs per squared centimeter, which typically provides good optical aesthetics. A high-density transplant of 40 to 45 FU/cm^2 is sometimes used at the frontal hairline to help improve coverage in select patients (ie, in a patient with high contrast between scalp color and hair color). In addition, the micrographs also include a small amount of skin and subcutaneous tissue, which actually extends the surface are of the recipient site and should be considered when transplanting (about 0.5–1.0 mm^2 on each graft). Other factors that impact the visible density of the hairs include the hair color, hair shaft size, color contrast between the scalp and the hair, and the presence of curl. These factors should all be considered and discussed with the patient during their initial consultation and during planning for their hair restoration.

SURGICAL PLANNING AND TECHNIQUE

Before the procedure, full photography is performed, including photographs of the patient from the front, three-quarter views, profile, occipital, vertex, and angled views looking right, left, and downward. It is important to carefully and thoroughly document the procedure because of the slow progress of the procedures. Often photographs of the proposed hairline can be performed, and additional photographs after surgery can also be performed. During the initial consultation, it is important to discuss the number of follicles to be transferred and also the likelihood of additional sessions based on the patient's prognostic factors for further loss.

POSITIONING DURING PROCEDURE

Positioning is of great importance when performing hair transplant surgery. The position of both the surgeon and the patient is helpful for comfort during the procedure for both parties. This procedure is performed under local anesthesia and, depending on the number of grafts and the patient, the surgical team could be working for 6 to 8 hours during larger sessions. It is of absolute importance to maintain comfort for both the surgical team and the patient to optimize the speed with which the procedure is performed. As both the patient and the surgeon can tire during the procedure, extra delays which lead to the local anesthesia wearing off, additional discomfort, followed by bleeding, and thus obscuring visualization and then further prolonging the procedure.

The strip can be harvested with the patient prone or seated upright. If the patient is prone, his or her head should be supported with a U- or O-shaped style frame to allow the patient to rest their head for the 30 to 45 minutes it may take to harvest the hair strip. The benefit of this positioning is that if the patient feels faint or may pass out, they are already lying down. In addition, this is the typical surgical position and so may be quicker and easier if one is used to this positioning. However, this then requires the patient to switch position to being seated and may require 2 separate pieces of equipment, an operative table for strip removal and a mechanical chair for the patient to be seated during site creation and hair placement.

The patient may also be seated upright during the harvest. With a mechanical chair that allows for the patient to be raised and tilted, this version of strip harvest permits the patient to remain in position for the creation of sites and placement of hairs. It also allows for a single chair to be used for easier positioning with less required movement. The downside is that if a patient feels faint, the procedure may have to be stopped to lay the patient down and elevate their feet. However, it reduces transitions needed during the procedure. Also, if entertainment is provided for the patient to watch, it can help distract them during the beginning of the procedure.

LENGTH AND WIDTH OF THE STRIP

The donor site is then prepared (**Figs. 1** and **2**). The site is prepared by clipping the scalp tissue to be harvested with a set of electric hair clippers. The

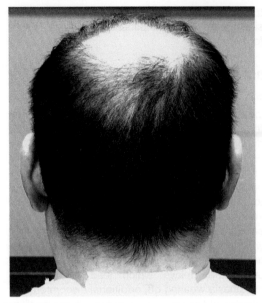

Fig. 1. Occipital scalp before preparing the donor site.

hair is clipped just to edge of what is to be harvested. The hair above and below the strip is kept intact so that there is immediate hair coverage of the scalp wound. The limits of the harvestable strip of donor scalp typically include the fringe scalp that is inferior to the occipital protuberance extending toward the ears bilaterally and below the line of maximal skull circumference.[3] Care should be taken to avoid excessive wound tension on the scalp wound. The scalp mobility should be assessed carefully. For patients

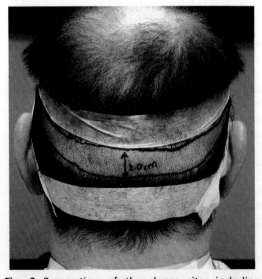

Fig. 2. Preparation of the donor site, including shaving the hair of the donor scalp and drawing out a strip to include approximately 3000 follicular units.

who have had a previous strip operation, the scalp excision can include the patient's previous scalp scar or can be placed in a separate location, avoiding the previous scar altogether. If a lower number of grafts are needed, the incision may be performed just on 1 side, leaving the contralateral side untouched for a future procedure.

The width of the strip is typically 10 to 15 mm but may extend up to 2 cm for larger cases (2500–3000 grafts). Care must be taken to ensure adequate scalp laxity because larger incisions may be a challenge to close in someone who has had a previous strip or with a very tight scalp. Significant tension on the scalp can result in a wide and visible occipital scar. The length should not go beyond the posterior aspect of the helical rim. The scalp skin adjacent to the mastoid is tightly adherent, and care must be taken not to go too low. The best hair density exists on the occipital scalp, but the lateral scalp hair is finer with more single hair follicles and so can be very useful during hair restoration, particularly for frontal hairline creation.[3]

SURGICAL EXCISION OF THE STRIP

Local anesthesia allows for patient privacy and independence because the patient may drive himself or herself to and from the procedure. Lidocaine (1%) with 1:100,000 epinephrine as well as small amounts of 0.25% Marcaine with 1:100,000 epinephrine are administered to the donor area using a 30-gauge needle. Once the donor site is anesthetized, additional tumescent (a standard Klein solution) can be injected into the donor site to help with both hemostasis and separation of the donor hair strip from the underlying subcutaneous tissue. Using a no. 10 blade with traction on the scalp, the skin is incised. Care must be taken to evaluate the directionality of the follicles while incising so that the surgeon does not inadvertently transect the follicles on the border of the strip. Once the skin and subcutaneous tissues have been incised, the lateral edge of the donor strip is grasped. With some tension and careful dissection, the subcutaneous plane can be quickly separated, avoiding occipital neurovascular injury (**Fig. 3**). No cautery is typically necessary unless the surgeon has inadvertently severed a deeper artery, which may require a ligature tie. A trichophytic closure of the donor site can be created by trimming a 1-mm strip of skin from the superior edge of the donor site. This trim can aid in creating an even narrower scar. Piercing towel clamps can be placed to help approximate the scalp tissues and allow for easy suture placement (**Fig. 4**). Because the scalp tissues are usually sufficiently lax, no undermining of the scalp

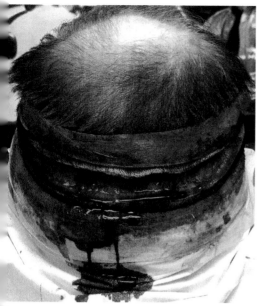

ig. 3. Removal of the strip has occurred. The subcu-
aneous tissues are visible, but bleeding is minimal.

ssues is usually necessary. Undermining is
voided if possible to avoid creating scar tissue
nat may affect future donor hairs. Closure typi-
ally can occur in a single layer with a running

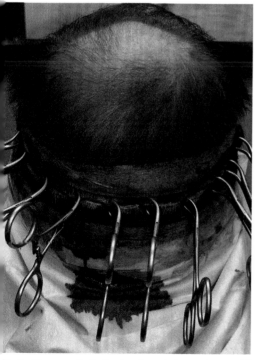

ig. 4. Placement of piercing towel clamps to provide
uick closure of the scalp wound and assist with rapid
uture closure.

3-0 polypropylene suture (**Fig. 5**). If there is significant tension, a 3-0 polyglycolic acid suture may
be used to close the deeper dermal layers. Staples
often are associated with more postoperative pain
because of having to lay on them for 2 weeks.
Once the hair is then cleaned and antibiotic ointment is applied, it is already challenging to detect
the posterior scalp wound (**Fig. 6**).

DONOR SCALP PROCESSING

Immediately following harvest of the scalp, the hair
is passed to the processing team (**Fig. 7**). Using
binocular microscopy (usually ×3.5) with a backlit
operating table, the strip is sectioned and slivered
into smaller sections. Using no. 10 blades, the
scalp slices are carefully prepared into follicular
unit grafts (**Fig. 8**). The micrografts (1 and 2 hair
grafts) and minigrafts (3 and 4 hair grafts) are
sorted. The micrografts are used for the frontal
hairline because they help better imitate the frontal
hairline. The grafts are kept on saline-soaked Telfa
sheets to prevent desiccation and reduced survival (**Fig. 9**). Ice blocks can be used under the
dishes to help keep the grafts chilled. It is imperative to maintain rapid, efficient coordination between the surgeon and the hair technicians to
decrease the amount of time that the grafts are
outside of the body. Studies have demonstrated
that graft survival begins to drop from 95% after
2 hours from harvest to transplantation to 86% after 6 hours to transplantation.[12]

RECIPIENT SITE CREATION

While the technicians are separating the strip, additional anesthesia is performed as a supraorbital
nerve block followed by injection along the hairline.
Additional tumescence is placed into the scalp tissues to provide hemostasis during site creation and
expand the scalp to allow the sites to be made
closer together and avoid the deeper neurovascular
structures. Under ×3.5 or ×4.5 magnification, site
creation is performed with 19-gauge needles. The
scalp is punctured to 4 mm deep to allow for placement of the grafts. The sites should be oriented with
the natural hairs. If the scalp is bare, the placement
should follow the normal angulation of the scalp,
which is typically 20° to 40° from the plane of the
scalp and more acute toward the frontal hairline.
In the medial scalp, sites are directed anteriorly,
and as the sites move laterally, they begin to be
directed more inferiorly.

PLACEMENT OF GRAFTS

After the site is created, the placement of the
grafts is then to be rapidly performed using

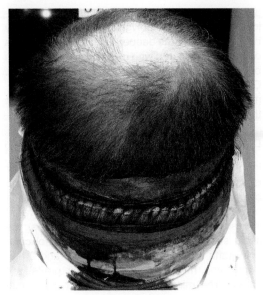

Fig. 5. Closure of the scalp wound with 3-0 running polypropylene suture brings together the hair-bearing tissue and tamponades any bleeding.

jeweler's forceps. Using multiple technicians, up to 3, can reduce out-of-body time for the grafts and help maintain their survival. During the site creation, the position, angulation, and depth of the graft were already determined, and so the grafts will find their way into the microincisions

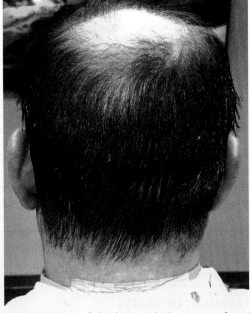

Fig. 6. Cleaning of the hair and placement of antibiotic ointment. Note that the incision site is challenging to detect.

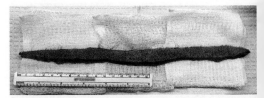

Fig. 7. Transference of the hair strip to the technician for preparation into individual follicular units.

as the surgeon intended. Initially the grafts are held in place by platelets and fibrin but are sealed in with tissue growth over the following week. It is normal for the hair shafts to shed in the following weeks or once the scabs have been removed. Although the hair shaft has shed, the follicular unit is still in place and will regrow the hair shaft. In addition, a telogen effluvium may also occur i the patient has existing hair that the transplant is occurring around. In that case, the patient may feel that they have less hair than they started with when the hair shafts shed. Often the patient needs reassurance during this portion of the healing process, and it is important to warn them about this preoperatively. Hair regrowth will then reoccur at 3 to 4 months postoperatively so that at around 9 months the patient should be seeing the final result with the transplanted hair indistinguishable from the native hair.

COMPLICATIONS

Complications from hair transplant are rare. Issues that may occur typically revolved around problems that may occur during local anesthesia-type procedures and can include bleeding, infection, numbness, vasovagal episodes, lidocaine toxicity, or anxiety. It is not abnormal for a patient to develop some periorbital swelling after the procedure from inflammation and use of tumescence. Postoperative

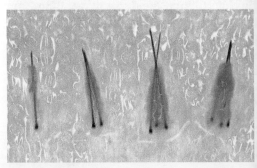

Fig. 8. Single, double, triple, and quadruple hair follicular unit grafts. (*From* Rawnsley JD. Hair restoration. Facial Plast Surg Clin North Am. 2008;16(3):290 with permission.)

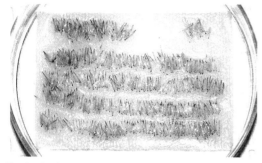

Fig. 9. Grafts are sorted into single and multiple follicular unit groupings with fine diameter singles set aside for hairline creation. (*From* Rawnsley JD. Hair restoration. Facial Plast Surg Clin North Am. 2008;16(3):295; with permission.)

treatment with a steroid can help relieve this issue. Erythema of the scalp recipient site will often resolve without any issue; however, it is important for the patient to avoid sun exposure to the site as well, which may worsen the erythema. If there are some buried grafts, a folliculitis can occur that may require unroofing with a needle but typically resolves without any intervention. Widening of the donor scar can occur from several of the issues mentioned above, including too much tension on the wound, strangulation from tight sutures, or follicular transection around the scar, leading to alopecia. As just mentioned, a telogen effluvium may occur at the recipient site or loss of some of the miniaturized hairs. Some of this loss may be permanent and may be shocking to the patient as well but was likely to occur naturally anyway.

Longer-term complications from hair transplant typically involve surgical planning missteps. Poor hairline planning, poor patient selection, and poor graft survival may all result in a suboptimal outcome. Graft survival can be impacted by long transplant times, mechanical damage, drying out of the grafts, exposure to excessive heat, or tissue ischemia. Poor hairline planning usually involves not taking into account future loss. In addition, using larger follicular units for the frontal hairline, poor angulation, and minimal microvariation at the hairline can lead to an unnatural-appearing result. Creating a too low of a hairline in a young patient can ultimately lead to hair gaps or a surgical appearance that may need to be corrected with further grafting. However, if that is not an option, laser hair removal may be needed to attempt to correct the improperly placed grafts.

SUMMARY

Follicular unit transplantation for hair restoration provides a natural, striking result while also allowing for short downtime and discretion for the patient. The aforementioned traits are all characteristics of the ideal cosmetic procedure. Men are often particularly sensitive to downtime, perioperative detectability, and effectiveness, and this procedure respects all 3 of these concepts. Success in hair transplant does, however, depend on proper patient selection and treatment planning. Creating a life-long hair restoration strategy with the patient is imperative to ensure a natural and long-lasting result in the face of the progressive nature of this condition.

DISCLOSURE

The author has nothing to disclose.

REFERENCES

1. Okuda S. The study of clinical experiments of hair transplantation. Jpn J Dermatolurol 1939;46:135.
2. Orentreich N. Autografts in alopecia and other selected dermatologic conditions. Ann N Y Acad Sci 1959;83:463.
3. Rawnsley JD. Hair restoration. Facial Plast Surg Clin North Am 2008;16(3):289–97.
4. Nordstrom R. Micrografts for the improvement of the frontal hairline after hair transplantation. Aesthet Plast Surg 1985;5:97.
5. Bradshaw W. Quartergrafts: a technique for follicular groupings. In: Unger WP, Nordstrom R, Rolf EA, editors. Hair transplantation. 2nd edition. New York: Dekker; 1988.
6. Headington JT. Transverse microscopic anatomy of the human scalp. Arch Dermatol 1984;120:449–56.
7. Cole J, Devroye J. A calculated look at the donor area. Hair Transpl Forum Intl 2001;11(5):150–4.
8. Bernstein RM, Rassman WR, Seager D, et al. Standardizing the classification and description of follicular unit transplantation and mini-micrografting techniques. Dermatol Surg 1998;24:957–63.
9. Rassman WR, Bernstein RM. The aesthetics of follicular transplantation. Dermatol Surg 1997;23:785–99.
10. Limmer BL. Elliptical donor stereoscopically assisted micrografting as an approach to further refinement in hair transplantation. Dermatol Surg 1994;20:789–93.
11. Rassman WR, Bernstein RM, Szaniawski W, et al. Follicular transplantation. Int J Aesth Restor Surg 1995;3:119–32.
12. Limmer BL. Micrograft survival. In: Stough DB, Haber RS, editors. Hair replacement: surgical and medical. St Louis (MO): Mosby; 1996. p. 147–9.

Follicular Unit Excision
Current Practice and Future Developments

Gorana Kuka Epstein, MD[a],*, Jeffrey Epstein, MD[a,b], Jelena Nikolic, MD, PhD[c]

KEYWORDS

- Follicular unit excision • Follicular unit extraction • Hybrid punch • Hair restoration surgery
- Hair transplantation • Follicular unit transplantation • FUE • FUT

KEY POINTS

- Follicular unit excision (FUE) is a safe and efficacious method of harvesting grafts with a low incidence of complications.
- There are a variety of devices that can be used for graft harvesting and they vary by the type and size of the punch, the method of penetrating the skin, and whether manual, motorized, automated, or robotic. The surgeon has options in picking the device that best suits his/her technique and skills.
- In the past 10 years FUE has gained in popularity due to rising patient demand because linear donor site scar remains and there is an easier recovery compared with the follicular unit transplantation (FUT) procedure.
- FUE remains a surgically more challenging procedure due to many components that have to be closely followed to have low transection of follicular units as well as ensure good healing of the donor area.

INTRODUCTION

Follicular unit excision (FUE) is a technique that has become popular in the past 15 years, and more surgeons are adopting this method as a preferable way to harvest grafts. It is a hair transplant technique where follicular units from the donor area are individually extracted using a punch 0.7 to 1.0 mm in diameter. This type of blind extraction was first described by Okuda in 1939[1] who was using punches of 2.5 to 3.0 mm diameter at the time, and it continued with the pioneering work of Orentreich[2] who was using a 4-mm punch, which is today considered the beginning of modern hair transplantation.

The first article about FUE was published in 2002 by Rassman and colleagues,[3] at which time the FUE technique was well defined but not practiced by most hair restoration surgeons. With the development of the technology and more accessible devices, followed by the interest of patients for this procedure, more physicians are now using this method to obtain grafts, and with growing experience they are getting faster and ensuring better quality grafts.

Instruments Available

The first tool used to harvest follicular units was a manual punch similar to the one used for skin biopsy. This sharp punch requires the surgeon to rotate it with thumb and index finger so that the punch penetrates the skin, then permitting the follicular unit to be extracted. Manual punch extraction is a slow and tiring procedure for the surgeon, and the trauma for the tissue is greater

a Dr. Philip Frost Department of Dermatology and Cosmetic Surgery, University of Miami, Foundation for Hair Restoration, 6280 Sunset Drive, Suite 504, Miami, FL 33143, USA; b Department of Otolaryngology, University of Miami, 6280 Sunset Drive, Suite 504, Miami, FL 33143, USA; c Medical School, University of Novi Sad, Hajduk Veljkova 3, Novi Sad, Serbia
* Corresponding author.
E-mail address: gorana.kuka@me.com

Facial Plast Surg Clin N Am 28 (2020) 169–176
https://doi.org/10.1016/j.fsc.2020.01.006

as the surgeon is rarely ever able to apply uniform pressure to the tissue.

This manual punch technique was been largely replaced, first by motorized devices, such as the SAFE system (Tiemann, Hauppauge, NY) and Ellis system (Ellis Instruments, Madison, NJ), which have the punch continually rotate. The surgeon can adjust the speed of rotation depending on the hardness of the tissue of the donor area.

Motorized devices are divided into 2 groups: rotating and oscillating, where the WAW system (Devroye Instruments, Brussels, Belgium) is the best known of the oscillating systems (**Fig. 1**). Here, the punch does not rotate in one direction, but rather oscillating back and forth, mimicking the use of manual punch. Finally, one of the newest FUE systems, Trivellini "Mamba" system (Buenos Aires, Argentina) uses a multiphasic drill system that includes a third type of motion, vibration, that theoretically further improves the dissection process.

There are also devices systems that have suction to help extract the grafts, such as the Neo-Graft (NeoGraft Solutions, Dallas, TX) and SmartGraft (Vision Medical, Glen Mills, PA). From the authors' experience and the observation of colleagues, the survival rate of the grafts harvested by NeoGraft is typically lower than that of some of the newer sophisticated systems, due to the potential for desiccation injury from constant air flow, as well as the use of less forgiving sharp punches combined with a rotary drill (see section Punches).

It is important to understand that 2 innovations in FUE systems have evolved in the past several years, and they involve different types of punches, as well as drills that deliver oscillating and even vibrating movement rather than just rotation.

The ARTAS system (Restoration Robotics, San Jose, CA) is the only robot manufactured exclusively for FUE. The device selects the FUs to be extracted, then the robotic arm makes the incision around the unit.[4] As with all of the other FUE systems described above, with the exception of NeoGraft and SmartGraft, which have a suction capability, every graft needs to be manually extracted from the site after the excision by the punch has been performed.

Donor Area Preparation

There are several ways the donor area can be prepared for undergoing FUE. The most common way is to trim the entire back and sides of the scalp, leaving the hairs in this total donor area at a length of 2 mm. This length is mandatory so the natural curve of the hair shaft can be followed during the FUE, yet short enough to permit ease in placing the punch over the desired FU. Another way to prepare the donor area for harvesting is to trim the hair down to 2 mm in "tunnels" along the back and sides of the head, each 2 to 3 cm wide, leaving the overlying longer hairs to conceal the trimmed hairs. This is very convenient, especially for female patients, but it imposes the risk of creating a so-called zebra effect due to horizontal rows of scalp that are thinned out from FU harvesting. A preferable alternative to trimming rows of hair is another form of "partial shave" FUE whereby the bottom 4 to 6 cm of the back of the head is trimmed 2 mm in length, appearing like an aggressive "fade," from which as many as 1200 to 1400 FU grafts can be harvested.

Finally, there are 2 options for doing a "no shave" FUE. The first way is an individual follicular trim isolation technique, first described by Harris,[5] trimming only those hairs that are going to be extracted. The other no shave FUE technique is "long hair FUE," whereby the individual FUs are extracted with the hairs left long, thus obviating the need for any trimming of hairs in the donor area. These no shave approaches are more technically challenging and time-consuming, but allow patients to have a fully presentable donor area immediately after. Another downside is that the total number of grafts able to be effectively harvested in a single procedure is typically 10% to 15% less than with a full shave, as less of the donor area is exposed for harvesting (**Fig. 2**).

Punches

There is a wide variety of punches that are commercially available, and they can be classified into 3 groups: sharp, blunt, and hybrid (**Table 1**). The extraction technique varies depending on the punch that is used. Sharp punches, the traditional punches used by many of the more conventional systems, have higher dissection properties and therefore the initial skin incision must be more superficial (around 2 mm) to avoid transection of the hairs. Blunt punches, first presented in

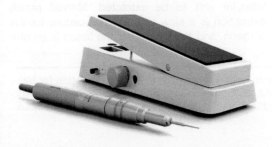

Fig. 1. WAW FUE system. (*Courtesy of* Devroye Instruments, Brussels, Belgium.)

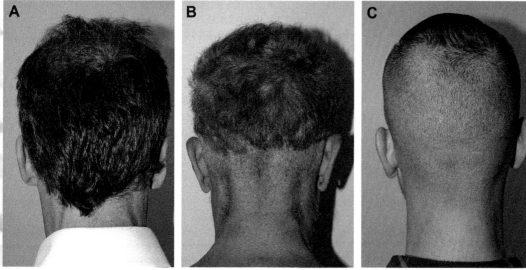

Fig. 2. Three ways to prepare the donor area for FUE: no shave (*A*), partial shave (*B*), traditional shave (*C*).

the Harris system avoid this risk of hair transection. The blunt punch needs to be introduced deeper into the skin (4 mm), and the punch may not cut through the outer skin as easily, which can result in a downward deforming pressure that alters the straightness of hair follicles being extracted. The hybrid punch is used in several systems, most notably the WAW and Trivellini and UGraft (Manhattan Beach, CA) systems. It uses some variant of a beveled outer sharp edge (to transect the skin) and an inner dull surface that atraumatically separates the FU from the surrounding adherent tissue, minimizing transection of hairs. Most of these hybrid punch systems use an oscillating rather than rotary movement, which is less traumatizing to the surrounding skin thus improving healing and reducing scarring. The Trivellini system has one type of hybrid punch that is designed to allow for the extraction of long hairs.

Our Technique

The safe donor area is marked out, and the surrounding zones above, below, and at the forwardmost temporal areas are also marked out as areas

of transition from dense to no harvesting (**Fig. 3**). These transition zones are critical to avoiding the "fringe effect," characterized as a dramatic contrast between the densely harvested donor zone and the surrounding areas. The safe donor zone is evenly

Table 1
List of available sharp, blunt, and hybrid punches

Sharp	Blunt	Hybrid
Cole serrated punch	Hex punch	Hybrid trumpet punch
Ertip punch		
Ring punch		

Table 2
Comparison between follicular unit excision and follicular unit transplantation method

FUE	FUT
No scalpels, no sutures	Wound edges closed with sutures and staples
No visible linear scar	Linear scar that can range from 1 to 10 mm wide
Shorter and easier recovery (healing time of 3–4 d)	Longer recovery (healing time of 10–14 d)
Up to 3000 grafts, 1–2 h of extraction	Up to 4000 grafts, 30–45 min of extraction
Other donor sites available (eg, beard, chest, abdomen)	No other donor sites available
Need to trim the entire donor area short, other than in an individual follicular trim method	Need to trim the donor area only where the strip is to be excised in the donor area
Higher cost in certain cases	Lower cost
Fewer assistants needed	More assistants needed

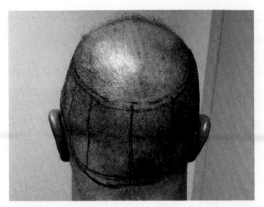

Fig. 3. Marking of donor area before FUE.

divided into marked out boxes to assure uniform harvesting. For example, if 1000 grafts are needed, the surgeon should extract 250 grafts per 4 boxes to ensure even harvesting, as shown in **Fig. 3**.

Anesthesia of the donor area is achieved first by a ring block with 2% lidocaine with 1:100,000 epinephrine, followed by the addition of tumescence consisting of 50 mL of saline, 10 mL of 0.5% bupivacaine, 0.5 mL of 1:1000 epinephrine, and 0.4 mL of triamcinolone acetate. Typically, to anesthetize the entire zone, a total of 20 to 25 mL of tumescence needs to be injected into the subdermal and deep dermal layers. Once the donor zone is anesthetized, with the patient in a prone position with his/her head resting comfortably in a specially designed pillow, the graft excisions may proceed painlessly, starting from the bottom right corner of the scalp (with a right-handed surgeon), proceeding cephalically and to the left in a specific pattern. As the surgeon moves forward with extractions, sufficient space is provided to the assistant for graft collection using 2 Forester forceps (**Fig. 4**). These grafts are placed into chilled storage solution, the exact type depending on surgeon preference. In our offices, we prefer Plasmalyte with ATP Solution (Thermo

Fisher Scientific, Waltham, MA) in petri dishes kept chilled.

Three aspects of excision are critical:

1. *Correct direction of the punch.* The visible 2 mm of the hair shafts emerging from the skin surface provide perfect guidance on ideal punch direction, angle, and positioning to assure the FU is in the center of the punch. Grafts that are more tightly packed with 2 and 3 or even 4 hairs are usually easier to be excised without transection of the FU. Curly hair, particularly in patients of African ethnicity, is more challenging to excise, as the curve of the hair must be mimicked with the motion of the punch.
2. *Correct depth.* The depth of the punch insertion varies on the type of punch. Sharp punches usually work best with more superficial penetration, no more than 2 to 2.5 mm to divide the attachment of the arrector pili muscle. Blunt and some hybrid punches work best with dissection to a depth of approximately 4 mm.[5] The only objection to this deeper dissection is a higher risk of buried grafts (around 7%).
3. *Proper pressure.* This pressure is applied to the donor area skin both by the surgeon's nondominant hand in the form of traction, and the actual punch. With introduction of tumescence, the skin becomes a bit tighter, potentially helping to achieve the ideal pressure with certain FUE systems. Excessive injection of the tumescence, however, might lead the donor area becoming mushy with lots of liquid underneath, making dissection more difficult. By applying pressure with the surgeon's middle and index finger above the FU to be extracted, the punch can enter the skin in a near-perpendicular angle, potentially reducing the diameter of the hole left after dissection, reducing scarring (**Fig. 5**).

Complications and How to Minimize Them

FUE hair transplantation is a relatively safe procedure associated with very few complications. Most of the complications are preventable with proper technique. One should remember that hair transplantation is a cosmetic procedure and any complication can have not only a cosmetic impact but also psychological outcomes for the patient, leading potentially to medicolegal implications.[6] All possible complications should be listed on the operative consent form. In our experience, the educated and properly consented patient not only is more compliant, but also has more confidence in the doctor due to the appearance of honesty and transparency.

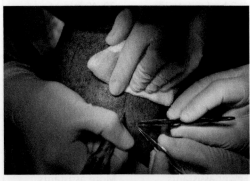

Fig. 4. Surgeon and assistant simultaneously doing FUE.

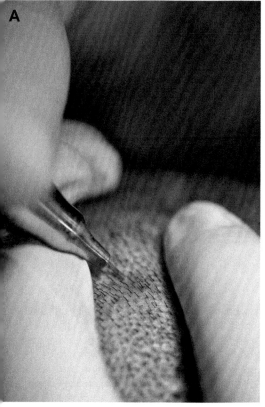 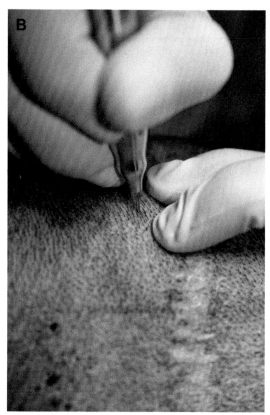

Fig. 5. Different angulation of the punch affects the scarring, as a more angled punch angle (*A*) leaves a larger punch hole than a more perpendicular angle (*B*).

Complications can be divided into those that are general for surgery and those that are FUE specific.

General complications include: adverse reactions to anesthesia, bleeding, tachycardia, syncope, and reaction to medications administered during and/or after the procedure.

Specific surgery-related complications include:

- Numbness in the donor and/or recipient areas
- Edema and swelling of the donor area
- Prolonged pain
- Infection
- Depletion of the donor area (moth-eaten appearance)
- Pinpoint scarring
- Buried grafts that can form cysts
- Alopecia areata
- Epithelial cysts
- Necrosis
- Hiccup or cough

FUE is a technique that avoids the appearance of the linear scar that results from the FUT procedure. However, if the FUE procedure is not properly planned, and the donor area is overharvested, the consequences are permanent. Detailed planning and thorough discussion with the patient will often minimize the rate of some potential complications.

Typical results demonstrate the consistent outcomes that can be achieved with FUE, with minimal risk of complications (**Figs. 6–8**). Regardless of whether grafts are obtained by the FUE or FUT technique, the key to achieving naturalness is the esthetic creation of recipient sites, the single most important aspect of the procedure in terms of esthetics. Having grafts that have consistent regrowth and implanting of these grafts into these recipients sites is essential, for only with these 2 components can the surgeon's vision of an aesthetic outcome be achieved.

Comparison of follicular unit excision and follicular unit transplantation

Because the FUE method found its application decades after FUT, it is to be expected that these 2 methods are going be compared (**Table 2**). However, these 2 techniques can also be successfully combined to maximize the use of the donor area and obtain the maximum number of grafts in a

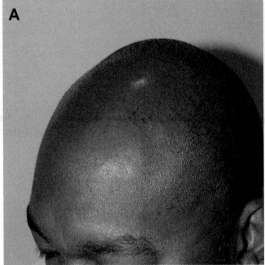
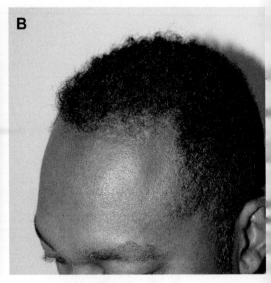

Fig. 6. Before (*A*) and 10 months after (*B*) 1750 grafts.

single session, when indicated, providing better coverage and density in patients with advanced degrees of hair loss. The "hybrid" approach, combining FUE with FUT, usually involves removing a single donor strip from the central back of the head, then, after suturing close the area of the strip, additional grafts from the surrounding safe donor areas are harvested by FUE, still respecting the borders of the safe donor area. Crisostomo and colleagues[7] described his method as "untouched strip" whereby he preserves a 15-mm-wide zone below his incision but above the zone of FUE.[7] This zone can be used in the future for another FUT procedure in select patients while preserving normal follicular density and avoiding fibrosis.

A major advantage of the FUE method is the absence of any linear scar on the donor area,

which permits patients to typically cut their hair short. However, with the rise of minimally supervised technicians doing this procedure and aiming for higher number of grafts while using bigger punches, there is a risk of permanent depletion of the donor area ("moth-eaten" or "barcode" appearance). The learning curve for FUE is steeper and therefore requires lots of practice to achieve excellence, but one advantage is that fewer assistants are required (1 or 2 is often sufficient) to do a case, compared with the typically larger team required to sliver and cut grafts with FUT.

In addition, the use of the FUE method opens the possibility of harvesting grafts from other hair-bearing zones, most commonly the beard but also potentially the chest, abdomen, and so forth. Although the body hair transplant grafts

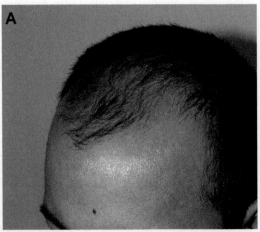
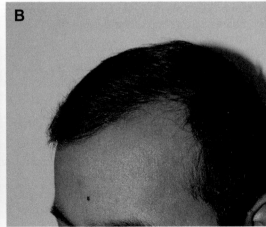

Fig. 7. Before (*A*) and 1 year after (*B*) 2050 grafts.

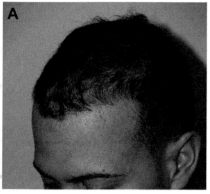
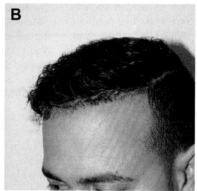
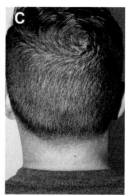

Fig. 8. Before (*A*) and 1 year after 1600 grafts showing hairline (*B*) and donor area (*C*).

night not be of the same quality, may have a different growth phase cycle, and can grow only to a certain length, this method can provide as many as 3000 or more grafts in selected cases (**Fig. 9**).

Controversies

As a relatively new procedure, FUE raises controversies, some ethical and some technical.

Who is doing the surgery?

Because in FUE there no use of typical surgical instruments, including blades and sutures, this has led to a minimalization of its complexity. Many entrepreneurs view this type of procedure as a perfect opportunity to make "easy" money with aggressive marketing, using nonmedical staff to perform the surgery. While using such deceiving terms, such as "non-surgical procedure," "minimally aggressive procedure," or "no-scar procedure," and overpromising the total number of grafts that can be safely transplanted in a single session, these clinics are attracting patients seeking to save money and maximize graft counts. Meanwhile, that high number of grafts is unrealistic in many cases, or to achieve requires overharvesting of grafts, including going outside of what is

considered the safe donor zone, resulting in permanent potentially visible scarring, to say nothing of poor esthetic outcomes due to the lack of surgeon involvement.

The position statement of the International Society of Hair Restoration Surgery (ISHRS) is that any procedure that involves tissue removal from the scalp or body, by any means, must be performed by a licensed physician, or similarly licensed Nurse Practitioner or Physician Assistant in Medicine (adopted by the Board of Governors ISHRS, November 15, 2014).[8] The term "extraction" seemed to be insufficiently surgical, hence the ISHRS changed the nomenclature of "follicular unit extraction" to "follicular unit excision" and defined "follicular unit excision" as consisting of 2 procedures: incision and extraction. In 2019, the ISHRS established a campaign named Fight the FIGHT (Fraudulent, Illicit & Global Hair Transplantation) to raise consumer awareness of the potential risk of having a procedure at a clinic where unlicensed physicians or technicians are doing the surgical aspects of the procedure—graft removal and creation of recipient sites.

It is the authors' opinion that harvesting tissue and creating recipient sites is the requirement of the surgeon, as these are surgical in nature, and

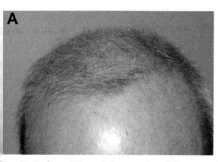
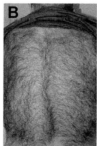
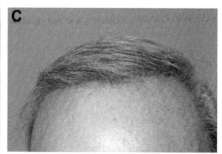

Fig. 9. Before (*A*) and 1 year after (*B*) more than 3500 FUE grafts harvested from the back (*C*) in an example of body hair transplant or body hair transplantation

that placing of grafts can be delegated to hair technicians who are trained to do it. This position requires the active intervention of state and national medical boards to protect the field from further issues that will discredit the FUE method, as well as to be in compliance of many states' laws dictating who can and cannot perform surgery.

Safe donor area

Definition of the safe donor area has been proposed by Unger and colleagues[9] where hairs in this area are androgen resistant and thought to be permanent. Larger FUE "megasessions" typically of more than 2800 grafts, have led to the need for grafts being harvested from larger parts of scalp, potentially into nonsafe zones. Some surgeons do harvest grafts from the nonsafe area after obtaining written consent from their patients who are aware that result is only going to be temporary. When promising FUE sessions above typically 2800 grafts, unless grafts have been divided, harvesting must often take place from the nonsafe area or too densely from the safe areas imposing the risk of donor area depletion.

Two methods—follicular unit excision and follicular unit transplantation: transection rates, quality of grafts, rate of regrowth

These 2 methods have been compared in so many ways, but ultimately it comes down to the quality of grafts. Initially, it was viewed that FUE harvesting can never meet the quality of grafts obtained by the direct-visualization afforded by strip dissection. With time, as more doctors started performing FUE and with the emergence of superior harvesting devices, there is essentially no difference in graft quality. FUE grafts can more easily emerge as "skeletonized," having a paucity of surrounding fat and tissue, and therefore are more fragile with a higher risk of poor growth. However, proper punch size choice, combined with surgeon experience, results in a significant decline in grafts that are transected or that are too skinny. African American patients do remain a challenge for the FUE method, but if the right motion is applied while excision around the follicle is performed, transection and partial transection of the graft can be avoided.

To compare FUE to FUT success, Josephitis and Shapiro[10] conducted a study in 3 patients undergoing a 2000-plus graft procedure, and compared graft yield, hair yield, and total graft and hair yield. The study results demonstrated essentially equivalent graft yields and hair yields per patient for both FUE and FUT.

Although a small study, this does provide evidence that FUE grafts are, at a minimum, not worse than FUT grafts, as thought years ago, and supports the enthusiasm of those who have helped advance FUE techniques.

SUMMARY

When they published an article on FUE for the first time in 2002, Rassman and colleagues[3] stated "FUE will find a role to play in hair restoration," and today, 18 years later, this method is becoming more popular and physicians are adopting it in larger numbers. Like any hair transplant procedure, proper patient selection (realistic goals, good donor supply) remains critical for achieving a good result, with FUE being very appealing to those who want to be able to cut their hair short after the procedure. Development of technology has helped surgeons to a great extent to be more efficient and obtain grafts of higher and higher quality while minimizing donor site scarring.

REFERENCES

1. Okuda S. Clinical and experimental studies of transplantation of living hairs. Jpn J Dermatol Urol 1939; 46:135–8.
2. Orentreich N. Autografts in alopecias and other selected dermatological conditions. Ann N Y Acad Sci 1959;83:463–79.
3. Rassman WR, Bernstein RM, McClellan R, et al. Follicular unit extraction: minimally invasive surgery for hair transplantation. Dermatol Surg 2002;28:720–8.
4. Avram MR, Watkins SA. Robotic follicular unit extraction in hair transplantation. Dermatol Surg 2014;40: 1319–27.
5. Harris J. Follicular unit extraction. Facial Plast Surg Clin North Am 2013;21:375–84.
6. Kerure AS, Patwardhan N. Complications in hair transplantation. J Cutan Aesthet Surg 2018;11(4):182–9.
7. Crisostomo MR, Crisóstomo MGR, Tomaz DCC, Crisóstomo MCC. Untouched strip: a technique to increase the number of follicular untis in hair transplants while preserving an untouched area for future surgery. Surg Cosmet Drrmatol 2011;3(4):361–4.
8. International Society of Hair Restoration Surgery. Available at: http://www.ishrs.org/. Accessed August 2, 2018.
9. Unger W, Solish N, Giguere D. Delineating the "Safe" donor area for hair transplanting. Am J Cosmet Surg 1994;11:239–43.
10. Josephitis D, Shapiro R. FUT vs. FUE graft survival: a side-by-side study of 3 patients undergoing a routine 2000+ graft hair transplantation. Hair Transplant Forum Int 2018;28:179–82.

Hair Transplantation for Scarring Alopecia

Anisha R. Kumar, MD, Lisa E. Ishii, MD, MHS*

KEYWORDS

- Scarring alopecia • Cicatricial alopecia • Inflammation • Platelet-rich plasma

KEY POINTS

- Scarring alopecia occurs when inflammation occurs at the upper hair follicle, destroying the associated stem cells and sebaceous gland.
- The key in treatment of scarring alopecia with hair transplantation is to first address the underlying disease process.
- There is a risk of reactivating the underlying disease process or having worsened hair loss when treating active disease.
- Potential complications specific to hair transplantation for scarring alopecia include ischemia, tissue necrosis, and infection.
- Platelet rich plasma can be used concurrently with hair transplantation to reduce inflammatory response.

INTRODUCTION

Hair loss can be a debilitating condition, especially for individuals who already have chronic underlying medical conditions that complicate the treatment of hair loss. Seven percent of patients in hair-loss clinics have scarring alopecia.[1] This article addresses the challenges pose by scarring alopecia in hair-loss treatment and the evidence-based practices that exist for hair transplantation in scarring alopecia.

SCARRING ALOPECIA

Also known as cicatricial alopecia, scarring alopecia occurs when inflammation occurs at the upper hair follicle, destroying the associated stem cells and sebaceous gland. The hair follicle is irreversibly damaged and replaced by scar tissue, thus leading to overall hair loss. Cases are also defined on the basis of predominant inflammatory cell type seen on biopsy: lymphocytic, neutrophilic, or mixed.

Scarring alopecia can be divided into 2 categories, "stable" and "unstable." Stable scarring alopecia occurs as a result of a single exposure or event, such as burns, trauma, radiation, or trichotillomania. Unstable scarring alopecia occurs in conditions that relapse and recur over time, such as lichen planus, folliculitis, linear scleroderma, and sarcoidosis.[2] Location of hair loss can also be particular to the underlying disease process; for example, central centrifugal cicatricial alopecia is most commonly seen on the scalp vertex, whereas frontal fibrosing alopecia typically affects the frontal hairline in a band-like pattern.[1]

Although clinical examination is the quickest and least invasive means of diagnosis, there is some discrepancy between diagnosis based on clinical examination and punch biopsy analysis, particularly with non-white patients.[3] While the gold standard for diagnosis is histologic analysis, newer techniques such as multiphoton microscopy (MPM) for the noninvasive visualization of

Department of Otolaryngology–Head and Neck Surgery, Johns Hopkins University School of Medicine, Johns Hopkins Outpatient Center, Johns Hopkins University, 601 North Caroline Street, Baltimore, MD 21287, USA
* Corresponding author.
E-mail address: learnes2@jhmi.edu

Facial Plast Surg Clin N Am 28 (2020) 177–179
https://doi.org/10.1016/j.fsc.2020.01.001

hair follicles are also allowing for less-invasive analysis of hair follicle size, sebaceous glands, and inflammatory cells in alopecia.[4]

CHALLENGES OF SCARRING ALOPECIA

Hair transplantation with scarring alopecia has unique challenges arising from the underlying disease processes. Factors to consider in assessing hair transplantation for scarring alopecia include donor hair availability, scalp laxity, the patient's healing patterns, vascular supply of donor and recipient region, and location of subsequent scar placement. Scarring alopecia affects the anatomy of the donor and the recipient hair regions. Hair grafts are less likely to take during an active disease state. Furthermore, even if the grafts take well, the underlying disease process can reactivate after the placement and can affect the longevity of the grafts. Additional potential complications more specific to hair transplantation for scarring alopecia include ischemia, tissue necrosis, and infection. Given these potential challenges, counseling patients and managing their expectations are extremely important. In addition to the graft possibly not taking, the hair transplant may result in sparse and fine hair and poor coverage, and outcomes may not be dramatic.[5]

OPTIONS FOR TREATMENT

The key in treatment of scarring alopecia with hair transplantation is to first address the underlying disease process. Patients with lichen planopilaris and frontal fibrosing alopecia had increased success in retaining transplanted hair after their disease was stabilized with treatment.[6,7] Underlying disease processes were treated with topical steroid cream, topical immunosuppressant cream, and intradermal steroid injection in combination with topical minoxidil and oral finasteride. To suppress underlying disease and prevent recurrent scarring, patients often continued with topical steroid treatment after the transplant.[6]

The Use of Follicular Unit Methods

The benefit of using follicular unit extraction rather than strip follicular unit transplantation has been shown in burn patients with scarring alopecia. The decrease in scalp laxity is a major consideration in choosing the method of transplantation, restricting the potential of strip follicular unit transplantation. Other challenges to consider in burn patients with scarring alopecia include the variable vascularity of mature scars and the impact on donor follicle survival.[8]

The Use of Whole Healthy Follicles

The importance of using whole healthy follicles in scarring alopecia has been demonstrated in patients with frontal fibrosing alopecia. After transplantation of healthy hair follicles, persistent follicular inflammation was seen at areas of preexisting frontal fibrosing alopecia, whereas the recipient sites of the whole healthy follicles did not have perifollicular inflammation. Because many of the underlying disease processes causing scarring alopecia involve an inflammatory reaction that leads to scarring, Scribel and colleagues[9] have theorized that inadvertently damaged follicles in hair transplantation may also express cytokines that trigger an inflammatory reaction of repair or apoptosis.

The Use of Platelet-Rich Plasma

Platelet-rich plasma (PRP) is a concentration for platelets 7 times the amount in normal plasma. Because the underlying disease process in scarring alopecia is inflammatory, PRP is another treatment option because of the various growth factors it contains, such as platelet-derived growth factor and vascular endothelial growth factor, which influence wound healing, tissue repair, and remodeling of scar tissue.

In one prospective randomized controlled trial that followed participants for 2 years, patients with androgenic alopecia who received PRP injections alone had increased mean number of hairs, mean hair density, epidermal thickness, and number of hair follicles 2 weeks after the last PRP treatment compared with patients who received placebo.[10] In another prospective randomized controlled trial, patients with androgenic alopecia who underwent hair transplantation and received intraoperative PRP immediately after the donor recipient sites were created had greater than 75% hair regrowth after 6 months; furthermore, activity in dormant hair follicles were seen in all 40 patients who received PRP while only in thirteen patients of the placebo group.[11] Furthermore, several case studies and retrospective review studies have shown that the use of PRP alone[12,13] and in combination with topical and intralesional steroids[13] improved the hair density of patients specifically with scarring alopecia.

SUMMARY

Scarring alopecia is hair loss secondary to underlying disease processes that create an environment of inflammatory response. Hair transplantation in this context is additionally challenging. The key to increasing the chances of success in hair transplantation for scarring alopecia is to treat the underlying disease process. Evidence-based options for transplantation exist, including use of follicular unit extraction rather than the strip follicular unit transplant method, ensuring the use of whole and healthy follicles to prevent further inflammatory reaction at recipient sites, and using PRP concurrently with transplantation.

DISCLOSURE

The authors have nothing to disclose.

REFERENCES

1. Filbrandt R, Rufaut N, Jones L, et al. Primary cicatricial alopecia: diagnosis and treatment. Can Med Assoc J 2013;185(18):1579–85.
2. Unger W. The surgical treatment of cicatricial alopecia. Dermatol Ther 2008;(21):295–311.
3. Zampella J, Kwatra SG, Alhariri J. Correlation of clinical and pathologic evaluation of scarring alopecia. Int J Dermatol 2019;58(2):194–7.
4. Lin J, Saknite I, Valdebran M, et al. Feature characterization of scarring and non-scarring types of alopecia by multiphoton microscopy. Lasers Surg Med 2018;51(1):95–103.
5. Parsley WM, Perez-Meza D. Review of factors affecting the growth and survival of follicular grafts. J Cutan Aesthet Surg 2010;3(2):69–75.
6. Liu YS, Shiou-Hwa J, Jung-Yi LC. Hair transplantation for the treatment of lichen planopilaris and frontal fibrosing alopecia: a report of two cases. Australas J Dermatol 2017;59(2):e118–22.
7. Cranwell WC, Sinclair R. Familial frontal fibrosing alopecia treated with dutasteride, minoxidil, and artificial hair transplantation. Australas J Dermatol 2016;58(3):e94–6.
8. Farjo B, Farjo N, Williams G. Hair transplantation in burn scar alopecia. Scars Burn Heal 2015;1. 2059513115607764.
9. Scribel M, Dutral H, Trueb RM. Autologous hair transplantation in frontal fibrosing alopecia. Int J Trichology 2018;10(4):169–71.
10. Gentile P, Garcovich S, Bielli A, et al. The effect of platelet-rich plasma in hair regrowth: a randomized placebo-controlled trial. Stem Cells Transl Med 2015;4(11):1317–23.
11. Garg S. Outcome of intra-operative injected platelet-rich plasma therapy during follicular unit extraction hair transplant: a prospective randomized study in forty patients. J Cutan Aesthet Surg 2016;9(3):157–64.
12. Saxena K, Saxena DK, Savant SS. Successful hair transplant outcome in cicatricial lichen planus of the scalp by combining scalp and bear hair along with platelet rich plasma. J Cutan Aesthet Surg 2016;9(1):51–5.
13. Dina Y, Aguh C. Use of Platelet-rich plasma in cicatricial alopecia. Dermatol Surg 2018. https://doi.org/10.1097/DSS.0000000000001635.

Platelet-Rich Plasma for Hair Restoration

Natalie Justicz, MD, Adeeb Derakhshan, MD, Jenny X. Chen, MD, Linda N. Lee, MD*

KEYWORDS

• Hair restoration • Platelet-rich plasma (PRP) • Androgenic alopecia • Growth factors • Hair loss

KEY POINTS

• Platelet-rich plasma (PRP) has been used to promote wound healing across a number of medical fields; more recently, the growth factor concentrate has become of interest for physicians interested in hair restoration.
• Androgenic alopecia (AGA) is a disease of progressive hair loss mediated by systemic androgens and other genetic factors; patients seeking PRP for hair restoration are commonly those with AGA who have not experienced success with finasteride or minoxidil.
• PRP is injected into areas of hair loss using a small-gauge needle, with most described techniques involving injections of small aliquots of PRP into areas of hair loss.
• PRP is a promising treatment for hair restoration in patients with AGA, and many studies of hair restoration with PRP report positive outcomes. Further research seeks to optimize PRP preparation/administration procedures and identify patient populations that benefit most from this treatment.

INTRODUCTION

Hair loss is treated with a wide range of clinical therapies including low-level laser light therapy as well as 2 medications approved by the Food and Drug Administration (FDA): topical minoxidil and oral finasteride. Surgical options include follicular unit transplant (FUT) and follicular unit extraction (FUE) techniques, which are outpatient procedures with excellent outcomes. In addition to these existing medical and surgical options, platelet-rich plasma (PRP) is a novel, minimally invasive, office-based procedure used to treat hair loss, typically secondary to androgenic alopecia (AGA). PRP consists of growth factors extracted from autologous blood obtained by venipuncture. This concentrated mix of growth factors is injected into areas of hair loss, stimulating hair regrowth.

BACKGROUND

PRP (sometimes called platelet-rich growth factors or platelet concentrate) was described in the field of hematology in the 1970s.[1] Hematologists coined the term PRP to describe a high-platelet product used for the treatment of thrombocytopenia. Within the fields of orthopedics and sports medicine, PRP has been shown to stimulate soft tissue and joint healing due to its high concentration of growth factors. Since the 1990s, PRP has been used to promote wound healing across a number of medical fields, including the following:

• Ophthalmology
• Oral maxillofacial surgery
• Cardiac surgery
• Gynecology
• Urology[2,3]

Department of Otolaryngology–Head and Neck Surgery, Harvard Medical School, Massachusetts Eye and Ear Infirmary, 243 Charles Street, Boston, MA 02114, USA
* Corresponding author.
E-mail address: linda_lee@meei.harvard.edu

Facial Plast Surg Clin N Am 28 (2020) 181–187
https://doi.org/10.1016/j.fsc.2020.01.009

More recently, PRP has become of interest to facial plastic surgeons, dermatologists, and those interested in its possible aesthetic applications and additional off-label uses.

According to the FDA, blood products like PRP fall under regulations set forth by the Center for Biologics Evaluation and Research, which regulates human cells, tissues, and cellular and tissue-based products.[4] Certain products, including growth factors like PRP, are exempt and therefore do not follow the FDA's traditional regulatory pathway (which necessitates animal studies and clinical trials).[4] Nearly all preparatory systems for PRP were designed to generate platelet concentrate to be mixed with bone graft material for orthopedic applications.[4] However, PRP is used for a wide range of off-label applications. Uses for PRP in the field of facial plastic and reconstructive surgery include the following:

- Soft tissue augmentation[5]
- Skin rejuvenation[6,7]
- Wound healing[8,9]
- Hair restoration

A review by Sand and colleagues[10] examined the early body of evidence for PRP in aesthetic surgery, including hair loss and facial rejuvenation. They concluded that PRP is a promising new therapy for AGA. One of the earliest articles on PRP for AGA was published in 2006 by Uebel and colleagues,[11] who described a 15% greater hair yield in follicular unit density in areas pretreated with PRP as compared with controls. This inspired interest and fueled the development of PRP technology for hair restoration and spurred its clinical adoption. A more recent systematic review paper by Chen and colleagues[12] examined PRP for hair restoration specifically in patients with AGA. Patient demographics, frequency of treatment, hair count, and hair density following PRP therapy were analyzed with promising results.[12] The hair restoration community is continuing to invest considerable time and resources in the development PRP therapies.

PLATELET-RICH PLASMA MECHANISM OF ACTION

Many growth factors have been identified in PRP, including platelet-derived growth factor, transforming growth factor-β, vascular endothelial growth factor, epidermal growth factor, and insulinlike growth factor. These factors are present in much higher concentrations (by a factor of 5 to 8 times) in PRP than in whole blood, and PRP has been shown to induce the proliferation of dermal papilla cells by upregulating fibroblast growth factor-7,

beta-catenin, and ERK/Akt signaling through these factors.[13] Although these growth factors are upregulated in PRP, the precise biological pathways by which PRP promotes hair restoration remain largely unknown. One proposed mechanism is that growth factors released from platelets act on the bulge area of hair follicles where stem cells are found, stimulating the development of new follicles and promoting neovascularization.[11,14]

PREPROCEDURE CONSIDERATIONS AND TESTING

Patients seeking PRP for hair restoration are commonly those who have not experienced success with finasteride or minoxidil for the treatment of AGA. AGA is a disease of progressive hair loss mediated by systemic androgens and other genetic factors. It is the most common type of hair loss for patients of both genders. AGA affects more than 73% of men and more than 57% of women by the age of 80.[15,16] As much as 58% of the male population between 30 and 50 years of age have AGA.[17] Many patients present to primary care providers, dermatologists, plastic surgeons, and otolaryngologists for counseling regarding hair restoration therapies.

As in any encounter leading to a prescription medication or procedural treatment, a full history and physical examination (H&P) are imperative for diagnosis of AGA. This H&P includes a detailed medical history, medication history, and clinical examination. Laboratory tests should be performed to exclude other causes of hair loss, such as anemia, malnutrition, and thyroid dysfunction. Labwork often includes a complete blood cell count, as well as a measurement of serum levels of iron, serum ferritin, total iron binding capacity, and folic acid. Thyroid function laboratory tests include T3, T4, thyroid-stimulating hormone, and antithyroid peroxidase. Other endocrine tests may include a measure of testosterone and other hormones. Autoimmune markers such as antinuclear antibodies may be examined. Some physicians, but not all, confirm the diagnosis of AGA with scalp biopsy. Once other medical causes of hair loss have been excluded, the patient and physician can consider the use of medications and treatments. Many patients with AGA start by trying FDA-approved medications. If topical minoxidil and/or oral finasteride do not provide significant improvement, patients become more willing to investigate more invasive procedures.

PRP does not take the place of hair transplantation via FUT or FUE. Rather, it should be considered in patients who may wish to stabilize hair oss or who are not ready to move forward with transplantation, acting as a standalone procedure to maintain or improve hair density and hair count. It also can be considered as an adjunct to hair transplantation.

Some additional contraindications exist when determining whether a patient is safe for PRP therapy. Patients with coagulopathies are generally not considered good candidates for PRP therapy and have largely been excluded from trials based on concern for periprocedural bleeding. Patients on anticoagulation or antiplatelet medications (such a clopidogrel or aspirin) also should be considered carefully, as they also may be at higher risk for bleeding. Moreover, as the mechanism of PRP may be related to the concentration and activity of platelets and platelet-derived factors, patients on antiplatelet medications were excluded from most studies to date, and therefore it is unclear whether they will see the same benefits. Reassuringly, a study within the cardiac surgery literature shows no statistical evidence of decreased growth factors delivered to the surgical wound site in the presence of aspirin and/or clopidogrel use,[18] but it is unclear whether this is generalizable to hair restoration treatments with PRP.

PLATELET-RICH PLASMA PREPARATION

PRP is prepared from a patient's autologous blood sample. A 18-mL to 30-mL venous blood draw yields 3 to 5 mL of PRP depending on the harvesting technique or preparation kit. There are many methods of creating PRP, but most have some steps in common. Blood is collected in tubes lined with anticoagulant, which are immediately centrifuged to separate the blood into 3 layers: red blood cells (RBCs) at the bottom, acellular plasma (PPP, platelet-poor plasma) is in the supernatant, and a buffy coat layer appears in the middle where platelets and leukocytes are concentrated in PRP (**Figs. 1** and **2**).[3] The subsequent steps vary between protocols as to which layers are harvested, but there is a general attempt to discard much of both the RBC layer and the PPP to collect only the material surrounding the buffy coat. After platelet-poor fluid has been discarded, the resultant platelet concentrate is applied to the surgical site. The time for platelet concentrate preparation can typically be completed in less than 1 hour.

PLATELET-RICH PLASMA ADMINISTRATION

PRP is injected into areas of hair loss using a small-gauge needle, such as a 30-gauge needle or an insulin syringe. Although PRP has also been used in the literature as a topical spray,[19,20] the vast majority of described techniques involve injections of small aliquots of PRP into the subcutaneous layer of the scalp. A local anesthetic, such as lidocaine, can be used, although most described techniques in the literature do not describe the use of a numbing agent. Lidocaine is not reported to disrupt hair growth, although this has not been well-studied. Alternatively, topical analgesia also can be applied as well as ice for vasoconstriction. In addition, the Zimmer cooler from a laser can be used during the injection for comfort.

Treatment areas can include the frontal, parietal, and occipital scalp. Typically, activated PRP is used, created by treating PRP with calcium chloride to activate platelets. Chen and colleagues[12] found that most studies used more than 1 treatment of PRP per patient, with most offering between 3 and 6 treatments with 1 month between injections. Patients should therefore be counseled to expect multiple rounds of treatment to maximize results.

POSTPROCEDURE CONSIDERATIONS

Few studies have noted any complications from PRP treatment. Some report temporary pain during injections[20,21] and transient edema/erythema at the injection site.[14,22] No allergic reactions, hematomas, or infections have been documented.

Patients can be counseled that there is no contraindication to showering or exercising following treatment. No antibiotic is needed. Most patients are able to return to work the next day. No significant or lasting swelling is anticipated.

PLATELET-RICH PLASMA OUTCOMES

Multiple retrospective studies, prospective trials, and systematic reviews suggest that PRP may be a promising new treatment for AGA. However, additional research is still needed to optimize the use of PRP for hair restoration.

The best use of PRP in terms of preparation, activation, and treatment regimens is unknown. Dohan Ehrenfest and colleagues[3] described a classification system of platelet concentrates based on preparatory process and leukocyte and fibrin content: P-PRP (pure PRP), L-PRP (leucocyte-rich plasma and PRP), P-PRF (pure platelet-rich fibrin) and L-PRF (leukoocyte-rich fibrin and PRF). Most published studies to date use an L-PRP derivate.[12]

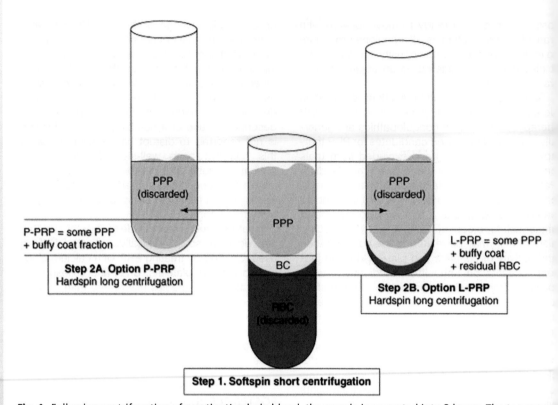

Fig. 1. Following centrifugation of a patient's whole blood, the sample is separated into 3 layers. The top supernatant component consists of PPP, and the bottom layer is composed of red blood cells (RBCs) or erythrocytes. The middle "buffy coat" (BC) layer contains the desired platelets and growth factors along with leukocytes. (*From* Dohan Ehrenfest DM, Rasmusson L, Albrektsson T. Classification of platelet concentrates: from pure platelet-rich plasma (P-PRP) to leucocyte- and platelet-rich fibrin (L-PRF). Trends Biotechnol. 2009;27(3):159; with permission.)

In the largest systematic review by Chen and colleagues,[12] 21 of 24 studies examining the effect of PRP on hair restoration reported positive outcomes (88%), both subjective and objective. Thirteen studies (54%) reported statistically significant improvement in at least 1 outcome that could be measured objectively. Hair counts or hair densities were described by 16 studies[14,21–35] and of these, 12 found statistically significant improvements in this outcome. Among studies with the highest level of evidence, 6 (75%) of 8 randomized controlled trials (RCTs) reported positive treatment outcomes. Three studies did not report positive findings after PRP administration, including 2 RCTs,[31,36] but these continued to report high patient satisfaction treatment results.

Future research should study the use of PRP in combination with minoxidil and finasteride. Most studies have excluded patients taking topical or oral medication within a certain period of study initiation (eg, 60 days or 12 months) so as avoid confounding results. However, for many patients it could make sense to try topical and oral medications in conjunction with PRP to maximize hair restoration potential. These patients would still be candidates for FUT and FUE hair transplant technology, which can be completed in conjunction with PRP therapy.

As patients with AGA can be affected at a young age, longer follow-up of patients is required to determine whether this treatment has long-lasting effects or whether repeated injections could be considered. In the literature, the shortest follow-up time for studies was 6 weeks and the longest was 1 year.[12] In addition, only 28% of patients in the systematic review performed by Chen and colleagues[12] were female; there remains limited information on potential gender differences in the effect of PRP.

The preponderance of evidence related to PRP and hair restoration is positive. It is becoming a more common procedure in hair restoration practices. Clinicians should familiarize themselves with the expanding repertoire of hair restoration treatments available to patients to provide individualized hair loss therapy.

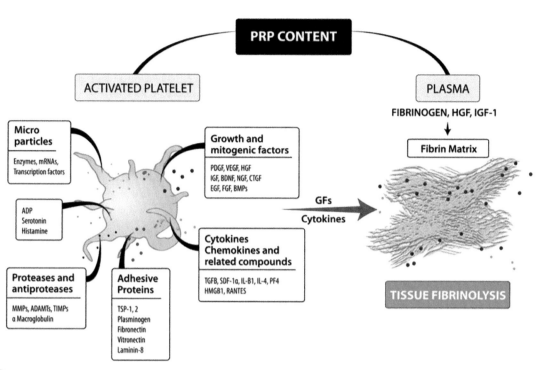

Fig. 2. Biological mediators of PRP that govern tissue repair by still poorly understood mechanisms. There are biomolecules and several growth factors that come either from platelet activation and plasma or both. Several of these bioactive mediators and other growth factors or proteins remain trapped through fibrin heparan sulfate–binding domains, in a 3-dimensional transient fibrin matrix to be released later by tissue fibrinolysis. ADAMTs, a disintegrin and metalloprotease with thrombospondin motifs; ADP, adenosine diphosphate; BDNF, brain-derived neurotrophic factor; BMPs, bone morphogenetic proteins; CTGF, connective tissue growth factor; EGF, epidermal growth factor; FGF, fibroblast growth factor; GFs, growth factors; HGF, hepatocyte growth factor; HMGB1, high mobility group box 1; IGF, insulinlike growth factor; IL-β1, interleukin-β1; MMPs, matrix metalloproteinases; NGF, nerve growth factor; PDGF, platelet-derived growth factor; PF4, platelet factor 4; RANTES, regulated upon activation, normal T cell expressed and presumably secreted; SDF-1α, stromal cell–derived factor-1α; TGFB, transforming growth factor beta; TIMPs, tissue inhibitors of metalloproteinases; TSP-1, thrombospondin-1; VEGF, vascular endothelial growth factor. (*From* Sánchez M, Garate A, Delgado D, et al. Platelet-rich plasma, an adjuvant biological therapy to assist peripheral nerve repair. Neural Regen Res 2017;12:47-52; with permission.)

SUMMARY

PRP is a promising treatment for hair restoration in patients with AGA. Created from a platelet concentrate from an autologous blood draw, PRP is a safe therapeutic option for patients with hair loss. It can be used alone or in conjunction with topical and oral therapies. PRP may also be administered before FUT or FUE.

Most studies of hair restoration with PRP report positive outcomes. Further research to optimize PRP preparation/administration procedures and identify patient populations that benefit most from this treatment are needed, in addition to long-term follow-up of objective hair loss outcomes. PRP appears to be a safe technology with excellent potential for promoting hair restoration.

DISCLOSURE

The authors have nothing to disclose.

REFERENCES

1. Matras H. Effect of various fibrin preparations on reimplantations in the rat skin. Osterr Z Stomatol 1970; 67(9):338–59 [in German].

2. Marx RE, Carlson ER, Eichstaedt RM, et al. Platelet-rich plasma: growth factor enhancement for bone grafts. Oral Surg Oral Med Oral Pathol Oral Radiol Endod 1998;85:638–46.

3. Dohan Ehrenfest DM, Rasmusson L, Albrektsson T. Classification of platelet concentrates: from pure platelet-rich plasma (P-PRP) to leucocyte- and platelet-rich fibrin (L-PRF). Trends Biotechnol 2009; 27(3):158–67.

4. Beitzel K, Allen D, Apostolakos J, et al. US defini-
tions, current use, and FDA stance on use of
platelet-rich plasma in sports medicine. J Knee
Surg 2015;28(1):29–34.

5. Ulusal BG. Platelet-rich plasma and hyaluronic
acid - an efficient biostimulation method for face
rejuvenation. J Cosmet Dermatol 2017;16(1):
112–9.

6. Asif M, Kanodia S, Singh K. Combined autologous
platelet-rich plasma with microneedling verses microneedling with distilled water in the treatment of
atrophic acne scars: a concurrent split-face study.
J Cosmet Dermatol 2016;15(4):434–43.

7. Shin M-K, Lee J-H, Lee S-J, et al. Platelet-rich
plasma combined with fractional laser therapy for
skin rejuvenation. Dermatol Surg 2012;38(4):
623–30.

8. Kang J-S, Zheng Z, Choi MJ, et al. The effect of
CD34+ cell-containing autologous platelet-rich
plasma injection on pattern hair loss: a preliminary
study. J Eur Acad Dermatol Venereol 2014;28(1):
72–9.

9. Sclafani AP, Azzi J. Platelet preparations for use in
facial rejuvenation and wound healing: a critical review of current literature. Aesthetic Plast Surg
2015;39(4):495–505.

10. Sand JP, Nabili V, Kochhar A, et al. Platelet-rich
plasma for the aesthetic surgeon. Facial Plast Surg
2017;33(04):437–43.

11. Uebel CO, da Silva JB, Cantarelli D, et al. The role of
platelet plasma growth factors in male pattern baldness surgery. Plast Reconstr Surg 2006;118(6):
1458–66.

12. Chen JX, Justicz N, Lee LN. Platelet-rich plasma for
the treatment of androgenic alopecia: a systematic
review. Facial Plast Surg 2018;34(6):631–40.

13. Gupta AK, Carviel J. A mechanistic model of
platelet-rich plasma treatment for androgenetic alopecia. Dermatol Surg 2016;42(12):1335–9.

14. Khatu SS, More YE, Gokhale NR, et al. Platelet-rich
plasma in androgenic alopecia: myth or an effective
tool. J Cutan Aesthet Surg 2014;7(2):107–10.

15. Hamilton JB. Patterned loss of hair in man: types
and incidence. Ann N Y Acad Sci 1951;53(3):
708–28.

16. Gan DCC, Sinclair RD. Prevalence of male and female pattern hair loss in Maryborough. J Investig
Dermatol Symp Proc 2005;10(3):184–9.

17. Krupa Shankar D, Chakravarthi M, Shilpakar R.
Male androgenetic alopecia: population-based
study in 1,005 subjects. Int J Trichology 2009;
1(2):131–3.

18. Smith CW, Binford RS, Holt DW, et al. Quality
assessment of platelet rich plasma during antiplatelet therapy. Perfusion 2007;22(1):41–50.

19. James R, Chetry R, Subramanian V, et al. Platelet-
rich plasma growth factor concentrated spray
(Keratogrow®) as a potential treatment for androgenic alopecia. J Stem Cells 2016;11(4):183–9.

20. Farid CI, Abdelmaksoud RA. Platelet-rich plasma
microneedling versus 5% topical minoxidil in the
treatment of patterned hair loss. J Egypt Women's
Dermatol Soc 2016;13(1):29.

21. Tawfik AA, Osman MAR. The effect of autologous
activated platelet-rich plasma injection on female
pattern hair loss: a randomized placebo-controlled
study. J Cosmet Dermatol 2017. https://doi.org/10.
1111/jocd.12357.

22. Anitua E, Pino A, Martinez N, et al. The effect of
plasma rich in growth factors on pattern hair loss:
a pilot study. Dermatol Surg 2017;43(5):658–70.

23. Kachhawa D, Vats G, Sonare D, et al. A spilt
head study of efficacy of placebo versus
platelet-rich plasma injections in the treatment of
androgenic alopecia. J Cutan Aesthet Surg
2017;10(2):86–9.

24. Rodrigues BL, Montalvão SADL, Annichinno-
Bizzacchi J, et al. The therapeutic response of
platelet rich plasma (PRP) for androgenetic alopecia
showed no correlation with growth factors and
platelet number. Blood 2016;128(22):2637.

25. Borhan R, Gasnier C, Reygagne P. Autologous
platelet rich plasma as a treatment of male androgenetic alopecia: study of 14 cases. J Clin Exp Derma
tol Res 2015;6(4). https://doi.org/10.4172/2155-
9554.10000292.

26. Gkini M-A, Kouskoukis A-E, Tripsianis G, et al. Study
of platelet-rich plasma injections in the treatment of
androgenetic alopecia through an one-year period.
J Cutan Aesthet Surg 2014;7(4):213–9.

27. Marwah M, Godse K, Patil S, et al. Is there sufficient
research data to use platelet-rich plasma in derma
tology? Int J Trichology 2014;6(1):35–6.

28. Sclafani AP. Platelet-rich fibrin matrix (PRFM) for
androgenetic alopecia. Facial Plast Surg 2014;
30(2):219–24.

29. Takikawa M, Nakamura S, Nakamura S, et al.
Enhanced effect of platelet-rich plasma containing
a new carrier on hair growth. Dermatol Surg 2011;
37(12):1721–9.

30. Gentile P, Cole JP, Cole MA, et al. Evaluation of
not-activated and activated PRP in hair loss treat
ment: role of growth factor and cytokine concentra
tions obtained by different collection systems. Int J
Mol Sci 2017;18(2). https://doi.org/10.3390/
ijms18020408.

31. Puig CJ, Reese R, Peters M. Double-blind, placebo
controlled pilot study on the use of platelet-rich
plasma in women with female androgenetic alope
cia. Dermatol Surg 2016;42(11):1243–7.

32. Gentile P, Garcovich S, Bielli A, et al. The effect of
platelet-rich plasma in hair regrowth: a randomized
placebo-controlled trial. Stem Cells Transl Med
2015;4(11):1317–23.

33. Alves R, Grimalt R. Randomized placebo-controlled, double-blind, half-head study to assess the efficacy of platelet-rich plasma on the treatment of androgenetic alopecia. Dermatol Surg 2016; 42(4):491–7.

34. Cervelli V, Garcovich S, Bielli A, et al. The effect of autologous activated platelet rich plasma (AA-PRP) injection on pattern hair loss: clinical and histomorphometric evaluation. Biomed Res Int 2014;2014: 760709.

35. Kang R, Nimmons GL, Drennan W, et al. Development and validation of the university of washington clinical assessment of music perception test. Ear Hear 2009;30(4):411–8.

36. Mapar MA, Shahriari S, Haghighizadeh MH. Efficacy of platelet-rich plasma in the treatment of androgenetic (male-patterned) alopecia: a pilot randomized controlled trial. J Cosmet Laser Ther 2016;18(8): 452–5.

Robotic Hair Transplantation

Marc R. Avram, MD*, Shannon Watkins, MD

KEYWORDS

- Robotic hair transplantation • Follicular unit • Elliptical donor harvesting
- Follicular unit extraction (FUE)

KEY POINTS

- Robotic hair transplantation allows rapid, accurate harvesting of follicular units from donor region with minimal scarring.
- Hair grows in natural 1- to 4-hair units on the scalp.
- Contemporary hair transplantation places natural follicular units from the donor region into thinning scalp in the frontal scalp, resulting in consistently natural appertaining transplanted hair.
- Elliptical donor harvest includes the cutaneous excision of hundreds to thousands of follicular that are then divided into individual follicular units by surgical assistants.
- Follicular unit extraction is the direct removal of natural 1- to 4-hair follicular units from the posterior scalp either manually, by device-assisted instruments or an independent robotic device.

INTRODUCTION

Hair transplantation has been performed for decades. It is based on the theory of donor dominance, which states that transplanted hair from the donor site (posterior scalp) will maintain its genetic destiny when you transplant into the areas of thinning in the frontal scalp (recipient sites).[1] From the 1960s until the 1990s, transplantation was a scientific success, but often an esthetic failure. The reason for this was that unnaturally large groupings of hair follicles were removed from the posterior scalp and placed in bundles of 10 to 30 pairs in the frontal scalp. This unnatural, pluggy appearance was cosmetically evident in many patients because hair naturally grows in individual 1- to 4-hair follicular groupings not bundles of 10 to 30 hair follicles.

In the 1990s, the concept of transplanting individual follicular units as opposed to multiple follicular grouping found in a pluggy transplant was introduced[2] (**Fig. 1**). This advance resulted in consistently natural appearing transplanted hair for patients (**Figs. 2 and 3**).

Donor harvesting techniques have evolved along with the size of the grafts. Elliptical donor harvesting involves excising a long narrow ellipse from the midocc.ipital scalp. The ellipse is carefully dissected into individual follicular units by trained surgical assistants using magnification to minimize transection of hair follicles.[3] The number of follicular units created depends on the density and size of the donor ellipse and the density and size of the recipient site to be transplanted. Elliptical donor harvesting is an efficient technique to harvest follicular units but it creates a linear scar of 10 to 20 cm in length. For the vast majority of patients, this scar historically was of no practical concern in the short or long term because their remaining hair in the posterior scalp camouflages the scar. For a minority of patients, particularly men who prefer short hairstyles, the scar could limit styling options.

Just as minimally invasive surgery has been gaining popularity in all of fields of medicine, in the early 21st century, the concept of follicular unit extraction (FUE) was introduced.[4,5] FUE was

905 Fifth Avenue, New York, NY 10021, USA
* Corresponding author.
E-mail addresses: mavram@dravram.com; michele@dravram.com

Facial Plast Surg Clin N Am 28 (2020) 189–196
https://doi.org/10.1016/j.fsc.2020.01.011

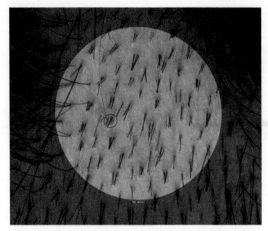

Fig. 1. Follicular grouping in posterior scalp.

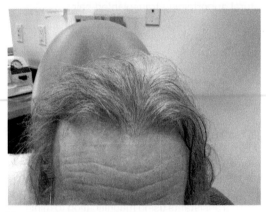

Fig. 2. Before hair transplant surgery.

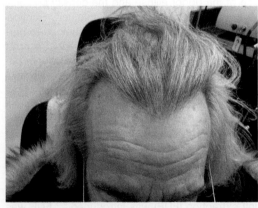

Fig. 3. After hair transplant surgery.

the direct harvesting of individual follicular units from the posterior scalp and then placing them into the recipient area in the frontal scalp. FUE allowed follicular units to be harvested without a single suture placed in the donor region. The

individual follicular units were harvested using 0.7- to 1.2-mm steel punches. The challenge fo physicians was the ability to efficiently harves many hundreds or thousands of individual follic ular units with minimal transection of follicula units. Transection of hair follicles can alter thei ability to grow. In some cases, transected hai will grow, but at a different rate and caliber thar the rest of the hair on the scalp. A variety of factors made the efficient harvesting of follicular units witI a low transection rate challenging including (1) the changing angle of growth of hair follicles within the scalp of a patient, and (2) operator fatigue fron prolonged hand–eye coordination when trying to efficiently remove follicular units with minimun transection of hair follicles. For some physicians manual FUE was a skill that could be learnec over time and for others this remained an ongoinç challenge. A variety of different instruments anc devices were developed to assist physicians witI extracting donor hair. Devices included custom made handheld punches, mechanical devices and suction-based devices (**Table 1**).

The goal of each device was to speed the ability of the surgeon to harvest large numbers of follic ular units.[6] What none of these devices did wa address long-term hand–eye coordination anc operator fatigue because, although each device helped to speed up the procedure, it did not main tain high quality with minimal transection of hai follicles.

In 2011, the US Food and Drug Administratior granted approval to the first true robotic device in dermatologic surgery (Restoration Robotics San Jose, CA). The robot was able to indepen dently choose follicular units and harvest them a the appropriate angle with minimal transection The challenge of hand–eye coordination and oper ator fatigue was eliminated. As with any instrumen or robot used in medicine, candidate selectior was vital to the success of the procedure. The robot is a technological marvel. Although truly ro botic by making independent decisions of where and where not to harvest hair follicles, the robo does not alter the need for appropriate candidate selection for the procedure. Studies confirm tha the robot is able to produce follicular units transac tion rates comparable to a skilled surgical team.[7,] This advance was a tremendous help for physi cians who did not have a trained surgical team.

- Transplanting individual follicular units as opposed to larger grafts made hair transplan surgery consistently natural appearing.
- Elliptical donor harvest has been and remains the state-of-the-art technique used in hai transplant surgery.

Table 1
Nonrobotic FUE

Device	Manufacturer	Details
Manual punches	Multiple different manufacturers	Size range from 0.7 mm to 1.2 mm
Motorized, Neograft	Neograft	A new, automated hair transplant system which facilitates the harvesting of follicles during a FUE hair transplant, dramatically improving the accuracy and speed over previously used manual extraction instruments.
Motorized, Smartgraft	Smartgraft	A suction-based system composed of a hand-piece, touchscreen monitor, and follicular unit graft storage chamber. During extraction, the SmartGraft system separates and counts the follicular unit grafts, and stows them in a sterile solution in the temperature controlled chamber. After extraction, follicular units must be manually placed into recipient sites that are created in the balding areas.
Motorized	Multiple different manufacturers	Motorized devices with punches to speed harvesting and reduce operator fatigue

- FUE is an alternative donor harvesting technique allowing minimally invasive surgery for hair transplant surgery.
- FUE has challenges regarding hand eye coordination, elevated transaction of hair follicles, and operator fatigue. The robot overcomes these challenges.

CANDIDATE SELECTION

As with all surgical procedures, candidate selection is the key to success for hair transplantation. Patients must have enough donor density in their posterior scalp to donate to fill thinning areas in their frontal scalp. The higher the donor density (follicular units/cm^2), the more hair available to transplant. The donor density for men and women does not always correlate with extent of hair loss in the frontal scalp. Regardless of a patient's density, all patients have a limited donor density available over a lifetime. This is the rate-limiting step of hair transplant surgery.

Both elliptical donor harvesting and FUE (robotic and nonrobotic) remain state-of-the-art donor harvesting techniques and should be discussed with patients as options (**Table 2**). Both procedures create individual follicular units that, when placed in recipient area, create natural appearing transplanted hair. For FUE, a patient's donor hair needs to be trimmed to 1 mm for harvesting whether performed manually or with the robot. For many men with shorter hair styles, this is a minor inconvenience that can be offset by the benefit of avoiding a linear scar. For most women and some men,

trimming their donor site hair to 1 mm is a major practical limit to pursuing FUE. In most women and men with longer hair styles, elliptical donor harvesting leaves a small linear scar that will be camouflaged by their hair.

Male and female pattern hair loss are chronic conditions with ongoing hair loss throughout life. The rate and extent of hair loss varies from person to person but it always continues. This concept is vital to review with all patients. The physician must plan for optimal short-term and long-term cosmetic results. A discussion of medical therapy to maintain existing hair is done for all patients. Minoxidil, low-level light laser therapy, finasteride (approved by the US Food and Drug Administration for men only), and platelet-rich plasma are all options that can be successful in helping to maintain existing hair. The risks and benefits of each treatment should be discussed in detail with patients (**Table 3**). It should be emphasized that the net perceived density from the procedure is equal to the amount of hair that transplanted minus the amount of hair that is lost through ongoing male and female pattern hair loss (net perceived density = hairs transplanted – hair lost via ongoing male/female pattern hair loss). Clearly, minimizing future loss through medical therapy allows maximum cosmetic impact from a hair transplant. A combination of successful medical therapy plus surgery will create the most perceived density from a procedure. The physician should always plan a procedure assuming a patient may want to stop medical therapy in the future and should consider how that would impact

Table 2
Robotic FUE versus elliptical donor harvesting candidate selection

	Robotic FUE	Ellipse
Donor scar	Pinpoint scars	Linear scar
Amount of donor region needing to be trimmed	Extensive. Difficult for women or men with longer hair. Not a problem for men with short hair styles	Minimal. Easy to camouflage for most women and many men.
Wound healing	4–5 d	7–10 d
Amount of donor hair available	Same	Same

the cosmetic appearance of the transplant. The frontal scalp for men and women has the greatest cosmetic impact with the fewest long-term cosmetic risk for most patients.

A patient's medical history should be reviewed. Certain medical conditions such as thyroid disorders, iron deficiency, and collagen vascular disease can exacerbate a patient's hair loss. Controlling them will help to slow further hair loss and may allow medical therapy to be more successful. It is important to review medications as well, because they may affect hair loss and/or the procedure. Preoperative and postoperative wound care and activities should be reviewed with patients (**Table 4**).

Patients should understand the finite amount of donor hair, the ongoing nature of male and female pattern hair loss, and how that will impact the density and cosmetic appearance of their hair over time. The ability to place hair where it will look natural in both the short term and the long term is also essential when determining whether a patient is a candidate for hair transplantation. As with all elective procedures, if a patient does not understand the limitations of the procedure it should not be performed.

- Candidate selection is key
- The majority of patients undergoing hair transplant surgery have pigmented terminal hairs remaining, pigmented hairs are necessary for the robot to function (however, can dye white hairs before the procedure and use the robot).
- Successful medical therapy is key for maximum long-term density after hair transplantation surgery and should be discussed with each patient during their consultation.
- Both donor elliptical harvesting and FUE should be discussed with all patients as donor harvesting options. For some patients, elliptical

Table 3
Medical therapy for male and female pattern hair loss

	FDA Status and Mechanism of Action	Potential Side Effects
Minoxidil (5% foam or solution)	FDA approved for male and female pattern hair loss. Mechanism of action unknown.	Irritation, dizziness palpitations, hirsutism, temporary shedding of hair with initial use.
Finasteride (1mg)	FDA approved men only. NOT women. 5 alpha reductase inhibitor.	Reversible sexual side effects, postfinasteride syndrome—can be long term off medication, gynecomastia, affect PSA/prostate cancer.
Low-level light therapy	FDA approved for men and women. Mechanism of action unknown.	Few side effects if used as directed by manufacturer. Visible light penetrates only into skin.
Platelet-rich plasma	Not FDA approved. No long-term safety/efficacy studies. Mechanism of action unknown.	Telogen effluvium. Medical clearance for patients with active medical conditions.

Abbreviation: FDA, US Food and Drug Administration.

Table 4
Preoperative and postoperative instructions

Preoperative Instructions	Postoperative Instructions
Review consent and written instructions sent to patient before the procedure. Anything unclear contact the office. Day of procedure eat/drink normally. Written consent/ verbal postoperative instructions reviewed. Area to be transplanted marked and photographed. The physician reviews the procedure with the patient.	Resume regular activities immediately. Avoid heavy exercise 5–7 d postoperatively. Prednisone 40 mg/ d for 3 d. Pain medication first 12–24 h. Overnight dressing removed next day. Shower day after surgery. Avoid picking scabs off. Let time/shower remove scabs over 5–8 d. Emollients to donor region twice daily for 5–10 d. Transplanted hair begins to grow 3–6 mo. Full hair growth 9–18 mo.

donor harvesting will be best choice, whereas for others FUE will be the best choice.

PREOPERATIVE PREPARATION

The procedure is performed under local anesthesia as an outpatient. Patients are encouraged to eat before they arrive, wear comfortable loose-fitting clothes, and bring any food, music, or video device they want to use during the procedure. We encourage all patients to let us know they need a restroom break or need to make a phone call during the procedure. Because the procedure takes hours, it is vital patients are comfortable and communicate with the surgical team. A relaxed comfortable patient makes the entire procedure easier for everyone in the room.

On the day of the procedure, the physician marks the area to be transplanted with the patient, and shows the patient to confirm both patient and physician agree on the area to be transplanted. Photographs are taken, and the patient is ready to begin the procedure.

- The procedure is performed using local anesthesia. Patients eat and drink before and during the procedure .

- The procedure and postprocedure wound care and activities are reviewed before the procedure and written instructions are given.
- The physician marks the area to be transplanted and confirms with the patient before beginning the procedure.

ROBOTIC FOLLICULAR UNIT EXTRACTION OPERATIVE TECHNIQUE

A combination of lidocaine and bupivacaine is used for the procedure. It is mandatory with robotic hair transplantation that the hair in the donor region is trimmed to 1 mm before the procedure is performed. The hair is trimmed to 1 mm by the surgical assistants using a moustache trimmer. Longer hair will prevent the robot from working at maximum efficiency (**Fig. 4**). The optical scanner of the robot used to identify and harvest follicular units needs to see pigment in hair follicles to function. Patients with gray, blonde, or red hair have the hair follicles dyed black by the assistants after being trimmed. This coloring is of no practical cosmetic impact because the hair is only 1 mm in length.

The patient lies in the prone position while the donor region is anesthetized. Once completed, the patient moves to the robot for donor

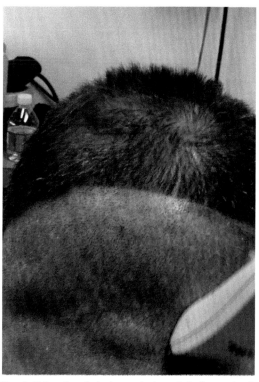

Fig. 4. Trimming hair 1 mm in length before robotic hair transplant.

harvesting. The patient sits in the chair designed for the robot with their head leaning forward and with their chin touching the top of their chest. This allows the robot to see and harvest the grafts optimally. A 3 × 3-cm grid is placed into the anesthetized area on the posterior scalp. This grid has fiducial markers to guide the robot to harvest follicular units within that grid. The robot calibrates and removes 90 to 110 follicular units from each grid (**Fig. 5**). Depending on the number of follicular units needed for the procedure 5 to 20 grids are used per procedure. The robot uses 2 punches— 1 sharp to cut through the dermis followed by 1 dull punch that then fires deeper into the superficial subcutaneous tissue to loosen an individual follicles unit from the skin. The robot has an algorithm that will not allow it to deplete a region on the scalp. The robot will not harvest grafts closer than 1.6 mm between follicular units (**Fig. 6**). Once the grafts have been created by the robot, a surgical assistant removes the follicular units and places them into a holding solution until they are placed into the recipient site. It is vital that the hairs do not desiccate. If they desiccate, they will not grow.

After the last follicular units are removed from the donor region, a temporary pressure dressing is applied to the scalp. The patient gets up

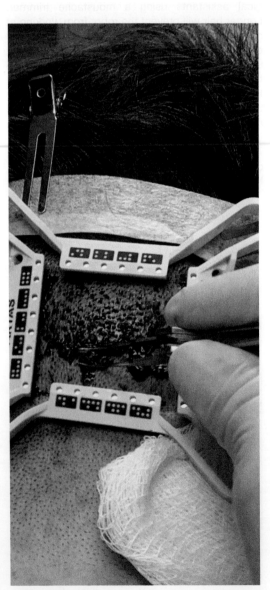

Fig. 5. Removing follicular units from grid using robotic technology.

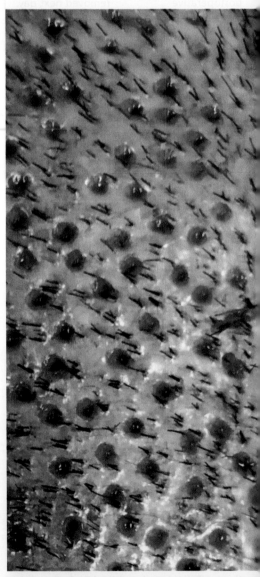

Fig. 6. Donor site after extracted follicular unit removed.

stretches, takes a break, possibly checking their messages or having a snack. After the break the patient returns to the room for placement of grafts into the recipient zone.

- Hair must be trimmed 1 mm and pigmented (if not it can be dyed) for the robot to work optimally.
- Local anesthesia is used throughout the hair transplant procedure.
- A 3 × 3-cm grid with fiducial markings to guide the robot is placed in the donor region. 80 to 110 follicular units are harvested within each grid.

CREATING RECIPIENT SITES AND PLACING GRAFTS

In addition to harvesting follicular units from the donor site, the robot is able to also create recipient sites and place grafts. However, using the robot to place grafts is less popular than using the robot to harvest, for several reasons. These include (1) the need to trim hair in the frontal scalp to 1 mm to make recipient sites and place grafts, (2) the robot is usually slower than a trained staff in placing grafts, and (3) there is less flexibility in creating custom hairlines than with a traditional 19G to 21G needle.

Many men will trim their posterior scalp for FUE, but many will be reluctant to trim their entire scalp to 1 mm for harvesting, site making, and graft placement. If there was a clear advantage for robotic placement of grafts in quality or speed, some would be willing to comply, but there is no clear advantage over a trained physician and surgical team in making sites and placing grafts manually with the current technology. Physicians or staff without experience in creating sites may find the robot helpful, but the robot offers no clear advantage for the patient in creating recipient sites.

Recipient sites created manually are done so with a variety of different needles or custom blades ranging in size from 19G to 21G. Sites are created at 30° to 40° angles parallel to existing hair follicles. Many physicians use magnified polarized LED lights for clarity and to assist in making recipient sites without transecting existing hair follicles. The surgical team then places the grafts using microvascular forceps.

- Recipient sites can be made manually using 19G to 21G needles or using the robot.
- With the robot, the hair follicles in the frontal scalp needs to be trimmed to 1 mm. This can be an impediment for some patients not wishing to trim their hair in the frontal scalp.

- Grafts can be placed manually using microvascular forceps or robotically. Hair needs to be trimmed to1 mm for the robot to place grafts.

POSTOPERATIVE WOUND CARE

Once the last graft is placed either robotically or by the surgical team, an overnight dressing can be placed. The dressing is to protect the grafts while they heal overnight. Patients can resume regular activities immediately, but are told to avoid strenuous exercise for 7 days. Patients can be given a short course of oral steroids to prevent frontal edema and a few pills of a mild pain medication. Unless medically indicated, antibiotics are usually not prescribed. The day after the procedure the dressing is removed by the patient and they can shower. Patients are then instructed to apply emollients to the donor region for 5 to 7 days. Patients can resume full sports and strenuous physical activities 1 week after the procedure. Postoperative perifollicular hemorrhagic crusting dissipates within 6 to 8 days with a daily shower. The transplanted hair enters a telogen resting phase 3 to 6 months after surgery. The hair follicles begin to grow 3 to 9 months after surgery and have a cosmetic impact for patients 9 to 14 months after surgery.

- An overnight dressing is applied after the procedure. Regular activities resume immediately. No heavy exercise for 1 week after the procedure.
- Dressings may be used, depending on surgeon preference. If used, they are typically removed the next morning. The patient showers and applies emollient over the donor region for 1 week. Perifollicular crusting in recipient sites disappears with daily showering in approximately 1 week.
- Transplanted hair grows 9 to 14 months after the procedure.

SUMMARY OF ROBOTIC HAIR TRANSPLANT SURGERY

Over the past 2 decades, men and women have been able to expect consistently natural appearing transplanted hair. This is due to the use of individual follicular units as opposed to larger grafts used in the past. The challenge for physicians performing contemporary hair transplant surgery is the ability to harvest and place hundreds to thousands of hair follicles during a procedure. To do this, a team of trained surgical assistants is required to efficiently perform the procedure. For physicians not performing the procedure regularly this was a difficult challenge to overcome. The robot is able to perform much of the work a trained surgical team would have done in the past. For some physicians this has been a revolutionary new tool.

The challenge remains appropriate candidate selection, realistic expectations, and successful medical therapy to maintain existing hair and planning a procedure for both potential short- and long-term future hair loss.

Furthermore, although the robot is a state-of-the-art instrument, it does not have the judgment and artistic ability of an experienced hair transplant surgeon.

- The robot allows surgeons without trained surgical assistants to perform hair transplant surgery
- The robot cannot tell the surgeon where to place grafts and where not to place grafts for optimal long-term cosmetic results.
- Candidate selection, effective medical therapy, and planning a procedure for both potential short- and long-term future hair loss are performed by the physician not robot

ACKNOWLEDGEMENTS

The authors thank Victor Masi (New York, New York, USA) for his help with the article.

DISCLOSURE

Consultant restoration robotics. Paid full price for machine. Pay full price for all consumables. No stock ownership.

REFERENCES

1. Dinh HV, Sinclair RD, Martinick J. Donor site dominance in action: transplanted hairs retain their original pigmentation long term. Dermatol Surg 2008;34(8):1108–11.
2. Bernstein RM, Rassman WR. The logic of follicular unit transplantation. Dermatol Clin 1999;17(2): 277–95. viii [discussion: 296].
3. Limmer BL. Elliptical donor stereoscopically assisted micrografting as an approach to further refinement in hair transplantation. J Dermatol Surg Oncol 1994; 20(12):789–93.
4. Rassman WR, Bernstein RM, McClellan R, et al. Follicular unit extraction: minimally invasive surgery for hair transplantation. Dermatol Surg 2002;28(8):720–8.
5. Avram MR. Hair transplantation: new concepts in 2005. J Cosmet Laser Ther 2005;7(2):77–80.
6. Garg AK, Garg S. Donor harvesting: follicular unit excision. J Cutan Aesthet Surg 2018;11(4):195–201.
7. Avram MR, Watkins SA. Robotic follicular unit extraction in hair transplantation. Dermatol Surg 2014; 40(12):1319–27.
8. Shin JW, Kwon SH, Kim SA, et al. Characteristics of robotically harvested hair follicles in Koreans. J Am Acad Dermatol 2015;72(1):146–50.

Hairline-Lowering Surgery

Jeffrey Epstein, MD[a,b,*], Gorana Kuka Epstein, MD[b]

KEYWORDS

- Hair transplantation ● Hairline-lowering surgery ● Complications ● Forehead reduction surgery

KEY POINTS

- Performed properly, hairline-lowering surgery has a low incidence of complications and very high patient satisfaction.
- Ideal candidates present with a stable frontal hairline and mobile scalp, as well as forward direction of hair growth to permit better concealment of the fine-line scar, and a goal primarily of forward advancement of the hairline rather than more rounding out.
- Although the design of the incision as explained in this article achieves some rounding out of the hairline, hair grafting may be performed as soon as 3 months after surgery if more rounding is desired. Hair grafting can also be used if indicated to help conceal any visibility of the scar.
- Primary risks for the complication of shock hair loss and scar widening are excess tension on the skin closure (which can be avoided by the securing the galea to the cranium), poorly executed galeotomies, and poor patient selection.

INTRODUCTION

Although not nearly as familiar as hair grafting to patients and physicians alike, hairline-lowering surgery (HLS) may be a preferable approach for lowering the overly high hairline, whereby on average more than 2 cm but as much as 5 cm of lowering can be achieved (**Figs. 1** and **2**), equivalent to transplanting as many as 7000 to 9000 grafts.

First described in the literature in 1999 by a plastic surgeon, Timothy Marten, who described forehead reduction with browlifting,[1] it has subsequently been written about as a standalone procedure[2,3] as well as in conjunction with frontal bone reduction.[4] In this surgery, essentially the entire scalp is advanced forward via a hairline incision with undermining in the subgaleal plane beyond the vertex, and secured in this advanced position using clips or other form of galea-to-cranium attachment, after which the excess forehead skin is excised and the incision closed. There are several key steps to ensuring optimal advancement and minimal complications, starting with proper patient selection, as described in this article. To ensure the best possible hairline appearance, a trichophytic frontal hairline incision, first described by Mayer and Fleming,[5] facilitates hair growth through the scar. The authors have performed 92 of these surgeries over the past 3 years, a dramatic increase in frequency attributable to both a greater patient awareness and enhanced confidence in the consistent results achievable through advancements in technique. Particular indebtedness goes to Sheldon Kabaker, whose modification to the technique provides a favorable rounding out of the hairline.[6,7]

PATIENT SELECTION

HLS is primarily indicated for shortening the genetically high hairline in women; however, it can be performed in the occasional male with a stable frontal hairline **Fig. 3**, as well as in the transitioning male-to-female patient in whom, if indicated, any prominence of the frontal bone and supraorbital rim can be reduced in prominence simultaneously.

[a] Department of Otolaryngology, University of Miami, 6280 Sunset Drive, Suite 504, Miami, FL 33143, USA;
[b] Philip Frost Department of Dermatology and Cosmetic Surgery, University of Miami, 6280 Sunset Drive, Suite 504, Miami, FL 33143, USA
* Corresponding author.
E-mail address: jse@drjeffreyepstein.com

Facial Plast Surg Clin N Am 28 (2020) 197–203
https://doi.org/10.1016/j.fsc.2020.01.002
1064-7406/20/© 2020 Elsevier Inc. All rights reserved.

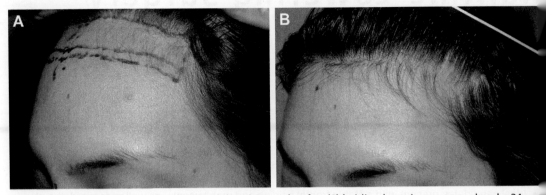

Fig. 1. A 22-year-old female patient, before (A) and 6 months after (B) hairline-lowering surgery whereby 24 mm of advancement was achieved.

There is no single parameter but rather 3 of them with regard to what constitutes the ideal hairline position. It can be located at a set distance of 7 to 9 cm above the nasion. Alternatively, it can be located along the junction of the vertical forehead and the horizontal scalp. Finally, the "rule of thirds" dictates that the upper one-third of the face should have the same approximate height as the lower and mid-thirds. These parameters primarily apply to the female hairline because a higher hairline is more readily accepted in the older male.

Many patients presenting for hairline lowering are requesting a shorter forehead—in particular, those who present to the facial plastic surgeon rather than the hair-restoration surgeon. Despite the specific request, it is not unusual that the patient in actuality is seeking a denser rather than lower hairline. In consultation the patient's specific goals must be determined, and the patient presented with the option, if appropriate, of hair grafting versus HLS. The first requirement for candidacy for HLS is a stable frontal hairline, without any risk of future hair loss caused by

male and/or female pattern hair loss. This is bes[t] determined by close examination of the fronta[l] hairs looking for the presence of vellus hairs, an[d] taking a good personal and family history of hai[r] loss. Progression of frontal hair loss will lead t[o] exposure of the hairline scar, and vellus hairs ar[e] at a higher risk of shock hair loss from the surgery[.] Because of this requirement, few men, particularl[y] those younger than 40 years, are appropriate can[-] didates for HLS.

The second requirement for candidacy is [a] reasonably mobile scalp that will permit suffi[-] cient hairline advancement. Mobility is evaluate[d] by placing 2 fingers directly behind the centra[l] frontal hairline and firmly pushing it forwar[d] observing the maximum amount of forwar[d] displacement possible (**Fig. 4**). There do no[t] seem to be any demographic factors associate[d] with good mobility, such as age, sex, or the de[-] gree (if any) of obesity, with the one exceptio[n] being of African ethnicity. The amount of forwar[d] displacement is a rough approximation of th[e] actual amount of lowering that will b[e]

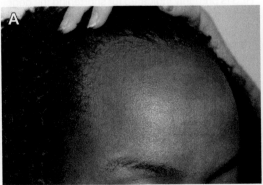
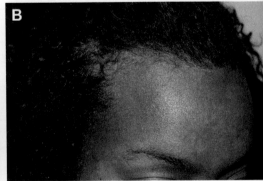

Fig. 2. A 34-year-old female African American patient before (A) and 6 months after (B) hairline-lowering surger[y] whereby 25 mm of advancement was achieved.

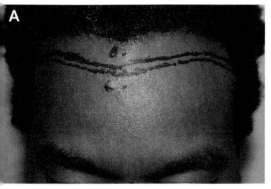
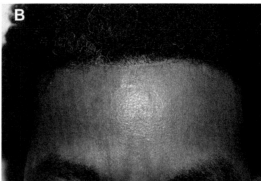

Fig. 3. A 42-year-old male African American patient before (*A*) and 4 months after (*B*) hairline-lowering surgery presenting for grafting to conceal the fine-line hairline scar. This patient had no risk factors for future male pattern hair loss.

achievable, knowing that an additional 3 mm of advancement on average will result from each of 1 or 2 galeotomies. It is noteworthy that in patients with limited scalp mobility, balloon tissue expansion can be performed; however, because this typically thins out somewhat the density of the frontal scalp and is fairly invasive, few patients are advised to undergo this procedure.

Contraindications for HLS include prior coronal or temporal browlift, temporal artery ligation, or any other condition that could compromise circulation to the frontal scalp. Prior hair transplant to the frontal region is not a contraindication, and in fact HLS can be performed to correct the inadequate density disappointingly achieved from a prior transplant. The patient should be seeking primarily a vertical shortening rather than a horizontal narrowing or significant rounding out of the hairline.

One indication for HLS that has undergone exploration is the management of the overly high hairline that has receded as a result of frontal fibrosing alopecia. Once this scarring alopecia condition has been controlled, the now higher frontal hairline can be safely advanced to a lower position, helping to reverse some of the recession that has occurred.

With HLS, the patient must be willing to accept what is a typically fine-line scar but has a risk of being visible, in return for the unsurpassed density of the lowered hairline and rapid results, in comparison with hair transplantation. The goal of this surgery is primarily lowering of the hairline rather than rounding out, whereby hair transplantation will be indicated. Finally, anterior direction of hair growth is preferable because it optimizes hair growth through the scar.

THE SURGERY

Before surgery, the incisions are marked out on the scalp. The first line runs along the existing hairline, just posterior to the vellus hairs that are too fine to effectively grow through the trichophytic incision. This line ideally should be somewhat irregular, extending laterally from the midline approximately 6 cm, then gently curving downward for approximately 1 cm to capture the frontalmost finer hairs of the upper temporal/frontotemporal junction, before making a right-angled turn and proceeding posteriorly in a horizontal direction for 1.5 cm. The next line is drawn to where the hairline can realistically be advanced, paralleling the irregularity and shape of the initial line (**Fig. 5**).

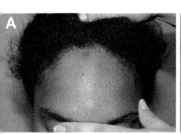
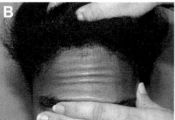
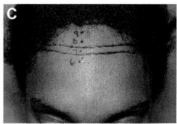

Fig. 4. Test of scalp laxity to assess how far the hairline can be lowered. (*A*) Before testing. (*B*) Displacement of hairline as far forward as it can be advanced. (*C*) Marking of the planned location of the lowered hairline.

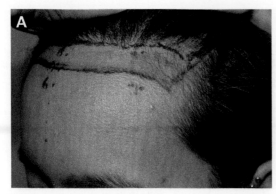
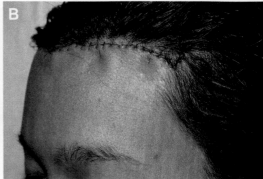

Fig. 5. (*A*) Two parallel incisions as described in the text, one along the hairline and the second to where it is anticipated the hairline will be advanced. (*B*) Immediate postoperative result.

Most of these procedures are performed under twilight sedation with local anesthesia, although oral sedation is typically possible. Lidocaine 2% with 1:100,000 epinephrine ring-block is performed, supplemented by supraorbital and supratrochlear nerve blocks. The ring-block should be sufficiently caudal on both sides and the back of the head beyond where the subgaleal dissection will extend. Tumescence with normal saline 40 mL along the hairline significantly reduces bleeding, avoiding the need for the injection of epinephrine, which can be associated with shock hair loss.

A trichophytic incision is made along the marked-out hairline, cutting through the follicles in a beveled fashion, then extending directly down to and through the galea to the periosteum. Scissors and blunt dissection undermine in the avascular subgaleal plane back to the vertex. This dissection is extended 2 to 3 cm beyond the vertex using a long endoscopic browlift dissector with Deaver retractor, optimizing visibility to facilitate cutting through the typically fibrous tissues that run between the galea and periosteum in this area. This dissection is similarly extended laterally to the upper temporal/parietal regions to optimize scalp mobility.

Once the undermining is completed, traction is applied to the frontal scalp using 3 towel-clips, firmly pulling the scalp as far forward as possible for 60 seconds. Two cycles of this mechanical creep are applied to the scalp to optimize forward displacement. Next, a coronal galeotomy is made approximately 25 mm posterior to the anterior edge of the frontal scalp, using a #15 scalpel blade to carefully cut through the galea and avoiding the vessels just above this layer (**Fig. 6**). Another cycle of mechanical creep is applied, typically obtaining another 3 mm of advancement. In most cases just a single galeotomy is performed, avoiding a

second galeotomy that increases the risk of shock hair loss.

The scalp is secured in its maximally advanced position using 2 clips, or any other method such as bone tunnels. The anchors of each of the clips are inserted into holes drilled into the cranium at a location each approximately 2 cm lateral to the midline, and positioned far enough anterior to where the hairline is intended to be secured. The small tines of the clips engage the galea of the maximally advanced hairline where it will hold the scalp forward in this desired position (**Fig. 7**). The clips will dissolve in 4 to 6 months, but the hairline will stay in place.

The excess forehead skin that overlaps the advanced scalp is then excised. Typically no undermining is performed into the forehead to avoid any elevation of the brows, unless a browlift is being combined with HLS. In this case, forehead dissection deep to the frontalis muscle can be extended to the supraorbital rims along with the desired management of the glabellar musculature, and this increased amount of skin is excised with the brows secured in position.

The hairline incision is then closed in a two-layer fashion, using interrupted 3-0 PDS sutures to approximate the frontalis muscle to scalp galea, followed by a running 5-0 nylon suture to reapproximate the skin edges. This is a trichophytic closure with the forehead skin overlapping the leading edge of the de-epithelialized frontal scalp. The temporal portions of the incision are closed with interrupted deep and skin sutures to work out any dog-ear deformity.

Antibiotic ointment to the incision and an overnight pressure dressing is applied. Patients are typically presentable on the very first day postoperatively, with either the hair brushed forward or a headband or cap covering the suture line. Normal hair washing and light exercise are resumed on the

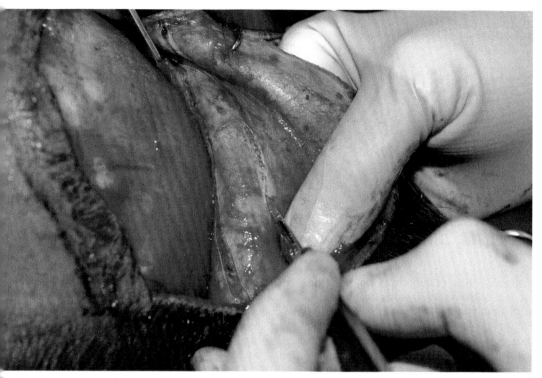

Fig. 6. Galeotomy is made with a #15 blade, keeping just to the galea to avoid transecting the more superficial vessels.

third day. Sutures are removed at 1 week, and by weeks hairs start growing through the scar. sensation to the frontal scalp, which has been disrupted by the hairline incision, in most cases starts to return by 3 months, with nearly every patient reporting full or near-full sensation by 6 to months.

COMPLICATIONS AND HOW TO AVOID THEM

Being a surgical procedure this, like any surgery that requires making an incision, carries a risk of scarring. Visible scarring can be due to one or more of several factors, including excess tension on the closure, inflammation and erythema, which is normal but can be associated with reaction to sutures or the hairs growing through the trichophytic incision, loss of surrounding hairs associated with impaired circulation or excessive tension, and finally poor healing resulting from both inherent factors and poor wound care. In general, most patients are content with the appearance of their hairline, and even among those who report some visibility of the scar this does not

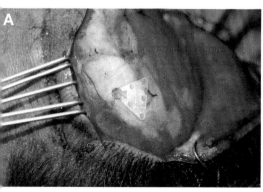
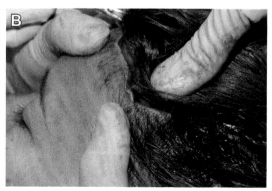

Fig. 7. One of the two clips is secured to the cranium (*A*), with the scalp then maximally advanced and secured to it (*B*).

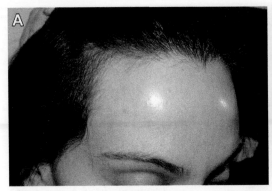
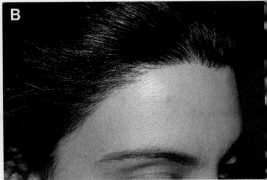

Fig. 8. A 31-year-old female patient before hairline-lowering surgery (*A*), then 18 months after surgery/14 month after hair grafting (*B*) to optimally round out the hairline and fill in the upper temporal regions.

seem to affect overall satisfaction with the procedure.

Although hair grafting can be performed to conceal scar visibility (see next section), it is always best to take measures to reduce its incidence. This includes avoiding skin tension at the closure by the use of clips to secure the scalp in position with pressure applied to the galea, and performing a proper 2-layered closure that has any tension applied to the deep tissue layer. Our experience is that 3-0 PDS is the deep suture that seems to cause the lowest incidence of reaction.

Steps to minimize hair loss at the incision line but also throughout the scalp include avoiding cauterization to the scalp, injecting no more than a small amount of 1:100,000 epinephrine to the hairline region, and careful creation of the galeotomy(ies). Saline tumescence is very effective in minimizing bleeding from incision edges, bypassing the need for any concentrated epinephrine beyond the 1:100,000 contained in the lidocaine in the ring-block. Tumescence also facilitates dissection through and reduces bleeding from

the fibrous bands connecting the galea to the peri osteum that are located at the posterior. In making the galeotomy incision(s), caution to avoid encountering the vessels that run in the immedi ately superficial layer to the galea will help ensure optimal circulation. What used to be a common approach of making 2 galeotomies has evolved into making just a single one in nearly all cases.

Despite taking these precautions, there will be some patients who experience hair loss after the procedure. However, the extent of this hair loss in the authors' experience falls far short of the extensive shock loss that is reported online, such severe loss likely being the consequence of poo surgical technique. The most common area o this mild hair loss in the authors' patients is along the incision, although in 2 patients it occurred overlying the clips.

HAIR GRAFTING

All patients at the time of consultation are evalu ated to determine the best approach: hair trans plantation or HLS. Those patients who meet the

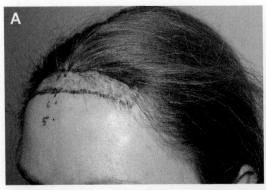
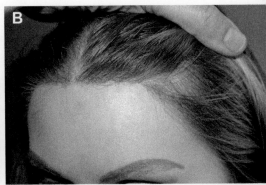

Fig. 9. A 27-year-old female patient underwent hairline-lowering surgery, shown before (*A*) and 4 months afte (*B*), to improve the disappointing results she had from prior hair grafting done elsewhere.

candidacy requirements for HLS (summarized earlier) are encouraged to undergo the procedure given the benefits over grafting, although most of these patients are advised that hair grafting may still be indicated. Grafting after HLS is appropriate for one more of the following: better rounding out of the hairline; softening and concealment if the hairline scar is at all visible; and further lowering of the hairline if desired, given the limited amount of lowering that in some patients can fall short of the ideal desired position.

Hair grafting is performed in approximately 50% of the authors' HLS patients. It is not advised to be performed simultaneously with HLS because of compromised hair regrowth and a limit on how close grafts can be placed to the hairline incision. Performed as soon as 3 to 4 months after HLS, a typical transplant procedure involves as few as 300 grafts for some rounding out of the hairline, to as many as 1500 to 1800 grafts to round out and conceal the hairline and possibly carry out further lowering (**Fig. 8**). These hair grafts can be obtained either by the follicular unit extraction or the strip technique, depending on surgeon and patient preference. To optimize regrowth along the hairline scar, platelet-rich plasma may be injected at the same time as the transplant.

SUMMARY

Hairline-lowering/forehead-reduction surgery has one of the highest levels of patient satisfaction in the authors' practice. The ability to achieve as much as 22 mm or more of lowering, along with some rounding out of the hairline, with the densest possible hair along with virtually immediate results, is a significant advantage over hair grafting (**Fig. 9**). With grafting, it can take as long as 10 to 14 months to fully realize the results, and in many patients who desire good density, a second smaller procedure is required to further fill in with more hair, requiring another 10 to 14 months to achieve the final result.

The trade-off is clear: a potential fine-line hairline scar and a more invasive surgical procedure (yet one that takes 2 hours or less to perform versus a 6- to 10-hour-long hair transplantation procedure of more than 2000 grafts) for a more rapidly achieved and unsurpassed dense hairline.

There are risks with HLS, however. Even in the experienced hair transplant surgeon's hands, hair grafting to lower the overly high hairline has limitations with regard to the density that can be achieved, as well as risks including prolonged erythema and superficial cellulitis or folliculitis. It would be interesting to objectively compare patient satisfaction achieved for each of these 2 procedures. Using the best-practice techniques summarized in this article, complications can be minimized and excellent outcomes achieved.

DISCLOSURE

The authors have nothing to disclose.

REFERENCES

1. Marten TJ. Hairline lowering during foreheadplasty. Plast Reconstr Surg 1999;103(1):224–36.
2. Guyuron B, Rowe DJ. How to make a long forehead more aesthetic. Aesthet Surg J 2008;28:46–50.
3. Ramirez AL, Ende KH, Kabaker SS. Correction of the high female hairline. Arch Facial Plast Surg 2009; 11(2):84–90.
4. Cho S, Jin HR. Feminization of the forehead in a transgender: frontal sinus reshaping combined with brow lift and hairline lowering. Aesthetic Plast Surg 2012; 36:1207–10.
5. Mayer TG, Fleming RW. Aesthetic and reconstructive surgery of the scalp. St Louis (MO): Mosby-Year Book; 1992. p. 121–4.
6. Kabaker SS, Champagne JP. Hairline lowering. Facial Plast Surg Clin North Am 2013;21:479–86.
7. Epstein JS, Kuka Epstein G. Surgical hairline advancement: patient candidacy and best techniques. Hair Transplant Forum International 2018; 28(5):184–6.

Hair Loss and Hair Restoration in Women

Samuel M. Lam, MD, FISHRS

KEYWORDS

- Female hair loss • Female hair restoration • Women • Hair transplant • Minoxidil

KEY POINTS

- Unlike for most men who suffer from male-pattern baldness, women should be thoroughly investigated for biochemical causes of hair loss as part of a standard workup before a hair transplant procedure should be considered.
- It is important for the surgeon to understand the clinical presentation of scarring alopecias, and the surgeon should have a low threshold to refer the patient for a biopsy to rule out this condition, which typically has a low success rate in hair transplant surgery.
- If a woman is deemed a safe candidate for female hair transplant, at times there is still limited donor capacity in the face of extensive global hair loss. Creative methods mentioned in this article, like designing T, L, and reverse L shapes, can be used to achieve good outcomes if the patient is willing to maintain a certain hairstyle.
- Female hair restoration should not be undertaken by the beginning hair surgeon owing to the complexity of the medical evaluation, the judgment on available donor hair for the degree of baldness, the risk of postoperative shedding, and the surgical difficulty of making temple and eyebrow recipient sites. However, if the beginning surgeon attempts only to perform limited central hair density improvements (and not hairline or eyebrow transplantation) in select women, then safe outcomes can be attained.
- Postoperative hair shock loss occurs in almost all women. Preoperative protection with minoxidil for a minimum of 6 weeks, extensive preoperative counseling, and methods to ameliorate the condition postoperatively should be well understood by the treating surgeon.

INTRODUCTION

Traditionally, hair restoration has been considered mainly a problem suffered by men. However, 30% of women over the age of 30 lose hair, and unlike men, who now socially can sport a shaved head, women do not have that option available to them. Full hair has been intimately tied with femininity and youthfulness, and hair loss in women can be psychologically even more debilitating at times than in men. In addition, female hair loss is oftentimes a much more complicated subject both medically and surgically speaking. Whereas oftentimes a man who presents to the clinic can be considered simply suffering from genetic male-patterned baldness, female hair loss may have a much more varied cause that demands investigation before a surgical hair transplant can be undertaken, if at all. In addition, there are nuances of surgery that must be understood to achieve excellent outcomes and requires a surgeon who is more advanced in the art of surgical hair transplant than merely a beginner. This article attempts to explore the many aspects of female hair loss and hair restoration in a highly practical manner for the surgeon and should serve as the beginning or continuation of a lifelong approach to the study of hair sciences.

Private Practice, Lam Institute for Hair Restoration, 6101 Chapel Hill Boulevard, Suite 101, Plano, TX 75093, USA
E-mail address: drlam@lamfacialplastics.com
Twitter: @drlam (S.M.L.)

Facial Plast Surg Clin N Am 28 (2020) 205–223
https://doi.org/10.1016/j.fsc.2020.01.007
1064-7406/20/© 2020 Elsevier Inc. All rights reserved.

facialplastic.theclinics.com

EVALUATION AND EXAMINATION OF FEMALE HAIR LOSS

Before surgical hair restoration can even be attempted, the surgeon must firmly grasp the eligibility of a particular female candidate. In addition, it is mandatory to evaluate in detail what could be causing this woman's hair loss and not simply assume that it neatly falls under the broad rubric of "female-patterned baldness." As mentioned above, the physician must serve as a sleuth fully to evaluate the patient's history, physical examination, laboratories, and if needed, even biopsy before considering surgery as an option.

Because female hair loss is a very large subject matter, it is worthwhile to try to simplify the clinical presentation to help guide a surgeon on a patient's management. While gathering the patient's history, dividing the type of female hair loss into stable and unstable can be instructive. If a woman reports that her hair loss is rapidly progressing, of recent onset, fluctuating in nature, constantly shedding, and so forth, surgery is almost entirely ruled out as an option until the disease process has been stabilized. In contrast, if the hair loss has been a slow, gradual loss over a period of many years with no abrupt recent episodes of shedding, then surgery could be an option. Nevertheless, it is imperative in women not to rush into surgery but to perform a careful and cogent analysis of the problem at hand.

If the woman complains of hair shedding, it is important to quantify how much hair she is seeing lost. Typically, 100 to 150 hairs a day can be considered normal, nonpathologic hair loss on days that she does not wash her hair with even greater numbers on days that she does wash her hair. The patient can be asked to count her hairs in the sink or shower and report back how many hairs have been lost each day over a period of time. It is also important to evaluate whether the hair has been actively shedding or just slowly being lost over time. The physician should also delineate the full nature of the hair loss: onset, causative agents, hair breakage, fluctuations, and prior treatments both medical and surgical for the hair loss.

Investigating a definable cause for the hair loss can also be helpful. For example, if a recent birth of her child, significant protein malnutrition/crash dieting, generalized sickness, general anesthesia, or similar, occurred approximately 6 to 12 weeks before the onset of hair loss, this type of hair loss could be caused by a condition known as telogen effluvium. Telogen effluvium is typically self-limiting and could be managed with minoxidil therapy until resolution. However, there is a condition in women known as chronic telogen effluvium in which they undergo repeated bouts of hair shedding and thinning over their lifetime. In contrast anagen effluvium occurs when there is an insul to the hair-shaft metabolism. For example chemotherapy or radiation can cause the hair shaf to break off and at times cause permanent hai loss. A history of chemical breakage or over hairstyling may also be elicited in trying to deter mine what is occurring.

It is important to inquire whether there are any other related symptoms that could be further fol lowed up using a biochemical evaluation or biops (both to be discussed later in greater detail). Fo example, if a young woman complains of heavie menses, iron deficiency is a very common caus for hair thinning and hair loss in women. If th woman has been steadily gaining weight and possibly experiencing thinning eyebrows, then hy pothyroidism could be a culprit. If menopause i settling in, then hormonal imbalances, such as an elevated dehydroepiandrosterone sulfat (DHEAS), could be a contributing factor. Th physician should inquire as to any scalp irritation such as burning, redness, flaking. These symp toms may indicate dermatitis on 1 end of the spec trum all the way to a scarring type of alopecia lik frontofibrosing alopecia (FFA) along with othe scarring hair losses. These conditions ma encourage the physician to have a dermatologis aid in the diagnosis through a targeted biopsy. I every case, a thorough history is the beginning c the investigation process.

Obviously, part of any history taking woul include prior surgical or traumatic causes for ha loss. For example, traction alopecia occurs pre dominantly in women of African descent who braid their hair so tightly that the hairs in the frontotem poral region are permanently lost (**Fig. 1**). This con dition is typically highly treatable with surgical ha transplantation. Prior brow lifting or facelifting ca cause alopecia along brow incisions and tempo ral/sideburn area and postauricularly (**Fig. 2**) Other traumatic injury and surgical incisions, fo example, neurosurgery, cancer reconstruction can also be sources for permanent hair los (**Figs. 3** and **4**). In general, with proper technique these types of hair losses may be corrected with hair transplant with consideration for the reduced blood supply from prior scar tissue.

As the history can be divided into stable and un stable categories, the physical examination can be simplified by grouping the disorders into patchy and patterned hair losses. In general, a patch type of hair loss may indicate a condition untreat able by surgery, whereas, in the right circum stances, a patterned hair loss could be surgicall

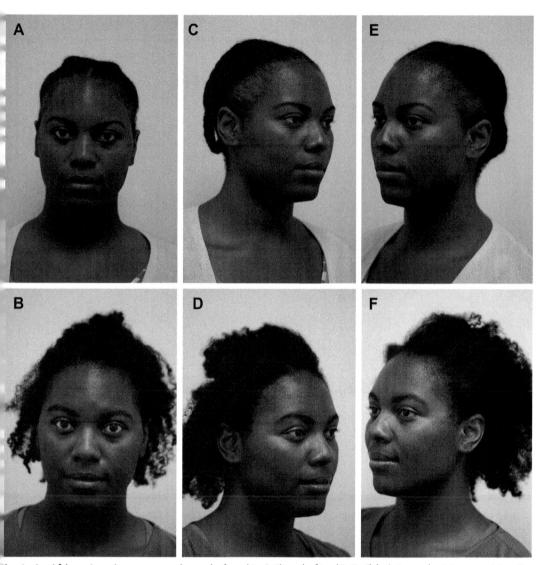

Fig. 1. An African American woman shown before (*A, C, E*) and after (*B, D, F*) hair transplant to correct traction alopecia. (*Courtesy of* Dr. Samuel M. Lam.)

managed. This categorization is overly simplistic but meant only to guide a physician's thinking so as properly to pursue further evaluation and to avoid operating on a patient who is an unsuitable candidate.

To understand a patchy type of hair loss better, it is wise to contrast this type of hair loss with standard female-patterned hair loss. Genetic female-patterned hair loss can be subdivided into 3 clinical presentations: Ludwig, Christmas tree, and a male-patterned appearance. Recognizing these types of female-patterned hair losses can facilitate a physician's ability to remark when a condition should deviate from a patterned hair loss. Ludwig hair loss involves a generalized thinning of the scalp hair that is graded from mild (1) to severe

(3) (**Fig. 5**). It can spare or involve the hairline, and the thinning can extend into the temporal, crown, and occipital regions. The Christmas-tree pattern described by Elise Olsen[1] may be considered a variant of a Ludwig pattern but is worth considering separately. When the hair is parted in the midline and viewed with the patient looking downward, the appearance of the hair loss resembles a Christmas tree with the base (the greatest loss) along the hairline/central forelock with progressively less hair loss posteriorly (the tree's apex) so as to resemble a triangular-shaped tree (**Fig. 6**). The final type of female-patterned hair loss essentially resembles male-patterned hair loss, usually owing to the hormonal imbalance that prevails at menopause. Studying the

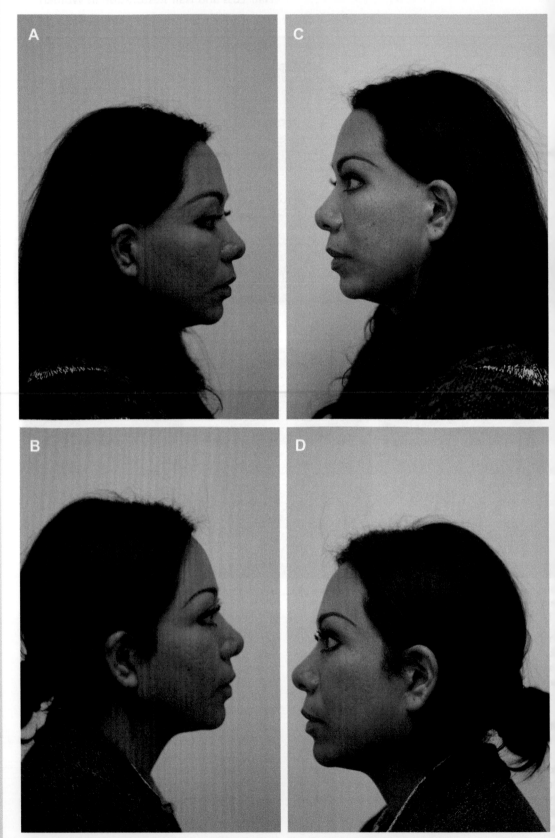

Fig. 2. A patient lost her sideburn and temple hair following a facelift, which was corrected by a single hair transplant session, and is shown before (*A*, *C*) and after (*B*, *D*). (*Courtesy of* Dr. Samuel M. Lam.)

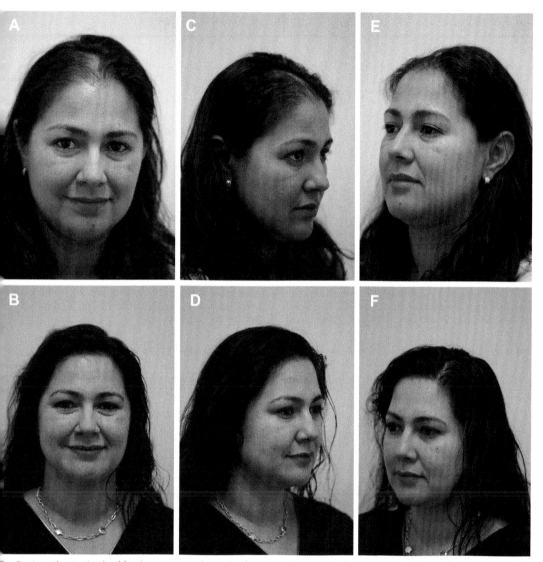

Fig. 3. A patient who had brain cancer and required surgery to remove the tumor and chemotherapy to address the cancer. She was left with hair loss from the chemotherapy and the surgery. She underwent a single hair transplant procedure and is shown before (*A, C, E*) and 10 months afterward (*B, D, F*). (*Courtesy of* Dr. Samuel M. Lam.)

Norwood-Hamilton chart for male-patterned hair loss can be a good start to understand how women also can similarly lose hair.

A patchy hair loss, on the other hand, describes a constellation of possible hair-loss conditions that are usually not amenable to surgery. If there is a patchy loss of hair that does not follow the above guidelines, it may represent other dermatologic/scalp conditions. For example, a painless circular area or areas of hair loss may indicate alopecia areata, an immune-mediated condition requiring steroid injections not surgery, or possibly trichotillomania. An inflamed or painful hair loss could indicate a scarring type of hair loss like central centrifugal cicatricial alopecia (CCCA), which is common in individuals of African descent, lichen planopilaris, discoid lupus erythematosus. If the hair loss represents a scarring hair loss, it can be considered a trichologic emergency because progression of this condition may lead to irreversible hair loss. Scarring alopecias, in general, do not do well with surgery and may either fail because grafts do not take or fail later when the quiescent disease reawakens.[2] In the past 2 decades, there has been a rising incidence of a scarring alopecia condition known as FFA that can resemble female-/male-patterned hair loss, and if transplanted, may lead to a failed surgical outcome. FFA presents clinically with progressive hair loss from the eyebrows upwards along the temples

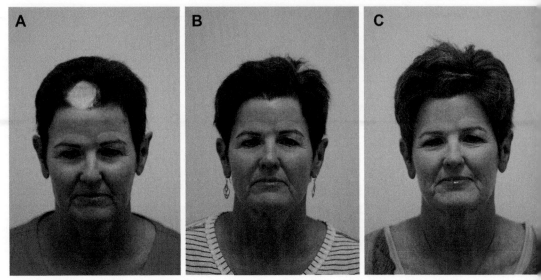

Fig. 4. A 59-year-old woman who is shown before (*A*), 1 year after having a hair transplant (*B*), and 5 month after having a second hair transplant (*C*). She wanted to replace hair in her scar after having a Mohs surger for skin cancer followed by a skin graft. (*Courtesy of* Dr. Samuel M. Lam.)

and may involve the entire hairline. There is typically a thinned and shiny appearance to the skin with a loss of pores, increased telangiectasias, and papules in the affected areas.

On physical examination, the physician mus carefully evaluate the pattern and extent of hai loss, the degree of miniaturization (conversion o thick terminal hairs into thin vellus hairs), alon

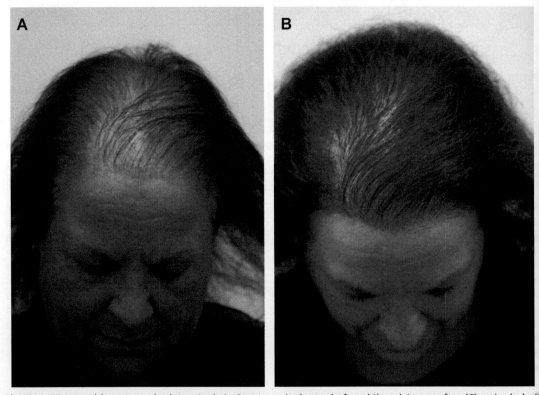

Fig. 5. A 55-year-old woman who has a Ludwig 3 pattern is shown before (*A*) and 1 year after (*B*) a single hai transplant procedure. (*Courtesy of* Dr. Samuel M. Lam.)

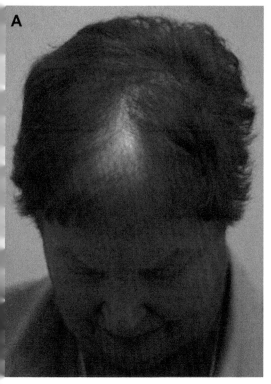 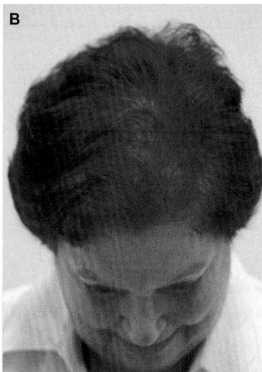

ig. 6. A woman with a Christmas-tree pattern of hair loss is shown before (*A*) and 1 year after (*B*) a single hair ransplant procedure to restore lost hair density. (*Courtesy of* Dr. Samuel M. Lam.)

vith any dermatologic disorders discussed above. There should be a low threshold for a physician to equest a biopsy if there is any suspicion of a dermatologic condition that would preclude surgery. When deciding on whether surgery would be a viable option for a patient, the ratio of useable donor hairs for transplant to the extent of baldness must be weighed. At times female hair loss can be so extensive as to involve not only the top of the scalp but also the entire donor region, making surgery ineffective because these transplanted vellus hairs will not provide much visual density and eventually be lost. This condition, known as diffuse unpatterned alopecia, is a contraindication to surgical hair transplant. Although follicular unit excision (FUE) can be used in women, follicular unit transplant (FUT) makes the most logical sense in most women who suffer from hair loss because the hair does not need to be shaved and for other reasons to be discussed in greater detail later in the operative section. Accordingly, scalp laxity should be evaluated either informally with finger manipulation of the occipital region or more formally using the Mayer-Paul laxity scale.[3]

In almost all female patients, it is advisable to perform a thorough biochemical evaluation, including iron, hormones (DHEAS, estrogen, testosterone, and so forth), thyroid function panel, erythrocyte sedimentation rate (and as needed an antinuclear antibody and other specific tests for autoimmune conditions), and a standard chemical and blood panel. If these studies are not already performed before the first consultation with the hair surgeon, the patient should be given the above list to be drawn by her primary-care physician and then to be optimized through medicine and/or bioidentical hormone replacement. In general, medical therapy targeted to a biochemical deficiency is important for long-term minimization of hair loss and partial reversal, but oftentimes it is insufficient in advanced hair-loss cases to fully reverse the condition. Surgery and medicine may work in a complementary fashion for the right candidate who would be suitable for both types of intervention.

Finally, as mentioned, biopsy can be a very important part of the evaluation for a patient suspicious of a dermatologic contraindication to surgery. Even a low suspicion of scarring alopecia should prompt the surgeon to seek the assistance of a dermatologist to rule out this condition that can imperil the success of a hair transplant procedure. In particular, what may appear to be traction alopecia could be in fact a scarring hair loss, because CCCA can mimic traction alopecia, especially if there is an obvious lesion in the vertex region. The unfortunate situation is that a biopsy is only as good as the dermatologist who performs it and acquires 4-mm sections for both horizontal and vertical sectioning in active regions of disease and is contingent also on the skill of the dermatopathologist who interprets the histology. If there is still a high suspicion after a questionable biopsy, it may be worth repeating the biopsy with perhaps another dermatologist/dermatopathologist. In addition, the surgeon who lacks a background in sophisticated scalp dermatology should spend the energy to research and learn about these conditions through textbook photographs and descriptions before embarking on a career as a hair surgeon.[4]

PREOPERATIVE CONSIDERATIONS FOR FEMALE HAIR TRANSPLANT

Once a woman is deemed safe and eligible for surgical hair transplant, it is then important to determine an effective operative plan that is well communicated to her in advance of the procedure and thoroughly documented in the medical records. In the electronic medical records, not only are a detailed history and physical examination completed but also a meticulous plan is completed of how many grafts to be harvested and in which areas those grafts will be transplanted. This information is recorded in a written narrative format as well as in a pictographic diagram in which the regions of the scalp planned to be transplanted are outlined and accompanying notes written on the diagram as needed for further clarification. On the preoperative visit when the patient meets with the nursing staff, hair transplant coordinator, and lead surgeon to sign and review consents and other documents, the diagram is reviewed again, and the patient signs off on the planned areas to avoid any miscommunication or finger pointing afterward. During the initial consultation or on the preoperative day, if a new hairline is to be planned (ie, not just restoring central density), standard photographic views are taken with and without the planned hairline drawn in using an erasable eyebrow pencil. These photographs are also entered into the formal medical record as a guide for the surgeon and as documentation for the agreed-on plan.

When deciding on an operative plan, there are several general considerations that a surgeon must contemplate that are different from those that apply to a man. First, no matter how thin a woman's hair becomes, she will not shave her head, unlike a man. Therefore, even restoring some hair density for her may be impactful, whereas in a man he may look better with a shaved head. Performing FUE or FUT is not scarless: the option for shaving one's head would be eliminated after any kind of hair transplant for a man. Second, no matter how thin a woman's hair becomes, women do not go completely bald, unlike a man. Accordingly, it is helpful to remember these 2 principles when working with women because if there is sufficient donor hair, some kind of hair transplant could be undertaken to provide some beneficial camouflage.

Despite these 2 relatively favorable dimensions to female hair loss, there are several issues that must be faced that are less ideal. First, women oftentimes lack sufficient donor hair because baldness can extend into the temporal hair-bearing area, relegating the surgeon to only harvest from the central occipital region. As mentioned, if the central occipital region also experiences thinning or miniaturization, this situation is a contraindication to hair transplantation. Furthermore, oftentimes the thinning is very global in nature, and there is a large area that must be covered with relatively poor donor hair capacity. If a woman has poor hair quality, that is, thin hair caliber, high hair color contrast to the scalp (eg, dark hair/light scalp or vice versa), lacks curl, or anything else that makes hair harder to achieve visual density when transplanted, then the odds of a successful hair transplant are further diminished. Unfortunately, many women have such global thinning that their donor hairs are compromised, and no hair transplant is possible.

Despite women having in some cases a poor ratio of limited donor availability to high recipient demand, the surgeon can uniquely design a transplant for a woman for optimal outcomes. Many women wear longer hairstyles than men and can use this flowing hair to camouflage other areas of the scalp that may not be transplanted. The 3 typical designs to restore female hair density are as follows: T, L, and reverse L (**Fig. 7**).[5] The goal is to restore the hairline/central forelock and the hair part. If the woman parts in the center, then the design would be a T. Similarly, if she parts on 1 side or the other of the head, then it would an L, where the vertical limb of the L would match the hair part. Oftentimes the hair loss can be so diffuse that trying to spread grafts over an entire scalp may lead to poor visual density. In many cases, it may be more advisable to strategize to focus on the most pertinent areas, as named above. Unfortunately, women would need to be counseled to adhere to 1 styling option based on the outlined surgical strategy. It is not to

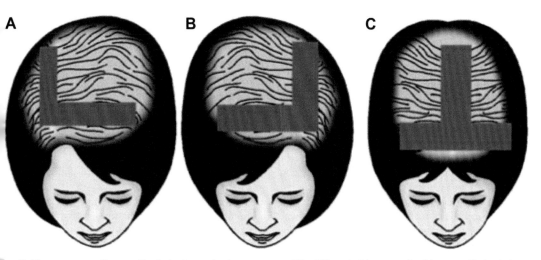

Fig. 7. Three prospective methods to transplant a woman with diffuse baldness and with more limited donor hair. (*A*) A woman who parts her hair on the right side can have the hair transplanted principally along the part and in the central forelock, an area behind the hairline. (*B*) A woman who parts her hair on the left side will have the mirror image of the L shape so that 1 limb falls along the hair part. (*C*) For a woman who parts her hair in the middle, an inverted T shape can be created so that 1 limb of the T falls along the central part. *From* Lam SM. *Hair transplant 360 for physicians, volume 1.* 2nd ed. Delhi: Jaypee Brothers Medical Publishers; 2015; with permission)

say that a woman always must have this kind of design: in a case where there is abundant donor supply and more limited loss, then a more global transplant can be undertaken. This decision-making process is part of the art of surgical hair restoration.

Another key preoperative consideration is medical therapy for female hair loss for a few reasons. First, if women are losing hair or continuing to lose hair, then medical therapy would be an important adjunct to a surgical option. Second, women in particular have a much higher risk of postoperative hair shedding that in the worst-case scenario may need to be camouflaged with a wig during the healing time. If there is even a mild degree of miniaturization of hairs in the area to be transplanted, a -week minimum course of minoxidil would be warranted to minimize postoperative hair shedding. In fact, perhaps it would be wise if all women were placed on this prophylaxis. All women are counseled preoperatively that they will have some degree of hair shedding; as the saying goes, an education is told beforehand and an excuse is the same words told to the patient but afterward. Education is far better than excuses. For women with mild shedding and some visible see-through, hair-fiber camouflage may be an inexpensive and simple solution until the hair grows back in in a few months. Creative hairstyling can also be used to cover any patches of hair loss caused by shedding. There are some intraoperative methods to further reduce the chances for

postoperative hair shedding, which are discussed later.

Minoxidil (5%) applied once daily for 6 weeks should be the minimum period of time that a woman needs this therapy before surgery, stopping minoxidil 2 days prior and resuming 1 week postoperatively. Women should also be counseled that they can show some shedding because the hairs are converted from telogen to anagen phase. It has been observed that a mixture of minoxidil with low-dose steroid (0.01% fluocinolone) and 0.01% retinoic acid may prove to be more efficacious in both men and women who suffer from hair loss than regular minoxidil.[6] If a woman develops any secondary hair growth, that is usually a good sign that the hairs will grow even better on the scalp, but if they want to back off, they could use 2% minoxidil. Low-level laser therapy (LLLT) has also been shown to be a good treatment but less effective than compounded minoxidil or standard minoxidil.[7] LLLT is applied 3 times a week for approximately 20 to 30 minutes each session. Platelet-rich plasma (PRP) has been less effective as a stand-alone therapy with at times excellent outcomes and on occasion less than stellar results. PRP can be used as a third treatment option for women following minoxidil and LLLT therapy.[8] There are also many types of supplement products that can help with hair shedding, but a full discussion of these products lies beyond the scope of this short article.[9]

OPERATIVE CONSIDERATIONS FOR FEMALE HAIR TRANSPLANT
General Principles

As mentioned, hair restoration for women is an advanced topic in terms of the medical conditions that must be understood and treated as well as the sophistication of the surgical treatments to restore female hair loss. There is a broad range of conditions that can be treated concerning female hair restoration, including female hairline lowering (for women born with high hairlines) (**Fig. 8**), traction alopecia repair, restoration of lost hair density, correction of postcosmetic surgery scars and hair loss following a brow lift and/or facelift, eyebrow hair transplant (**Fig. 9**), and reconstructive hair transplant for chemotherapy, radiation, cancer, trauma, and so on. These conditions are just some of the representative conditions that a surgeon can treat for women suffering from hair loss. Of course, there are also transgender patients who are women transitioning to become men wanting facial hair transplants, or, more commonly, men transitioning to women who want a female hairline and hair density. This last

topic lies beyond what this article describes. This section outlines first some general ideas of donor harvesting and recipient-site creation that are relevant for female hair transplant and then briefly outlines techniques for each of the above-stated conditions. This article does not offer a step-by-step how-to hair transplant guide but focuses on salient concerns for the surgeon when he or she treats a female patient for surgical hair restoration.

Anesthesia Considerations

One of the most dreaded concerns that plague a surgeon operating on a woman for hair loss is postoperative hair shock loss. Most times, this condition is only temporary, but at times, the hair may not fully return. As mentioned, use of 5% minoxidil along with other treatment options, like LLLT or oral supplements, should be used to minimize this risk for a minimum of 6 weeks preoperatively. Beyond this treatment, there are some intraoperative anesthesia considerations that can help minimize postoperative shock loss. Reduction of the epinephrine load to the patient has been thought to limit the risk of shock loss

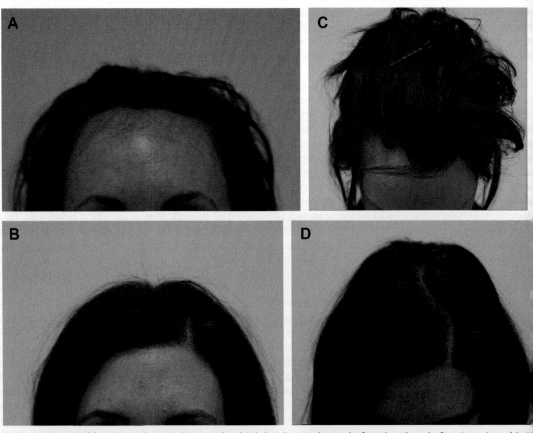

Fig. 8. A 29-year-old patient who was born with a high hairline is shown before (*A, B*) and after 2 sessions (*C, D*) of hair transplantation to lower her hairline. (*Courtesy of* Dr. Samuel M. Lam.)

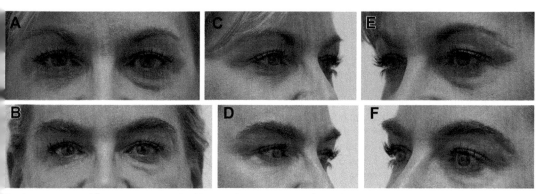

Fig. 9. A 50-year-old woman overplucked her eyebrows, leaving them thin and unattractive. She is shown before (A, C, E) and 5 months after (B, D, F) a single eyebrow hair transplant procedure. (*Courtesy of* Dr. Samuel M. Lam.)

because the epinephrine may create excessive vasoconstriction, which in turn may promote postoperative hair loss. For the circumferential ring block, the same anesthetic is used for both men and women, namely, initially 1% lidocaine with 1:100,000 epinephrine followed by 0.25% bupivacaine with 1:200,000 epinephrine. However, for the donor and recipient tumescent anesthesia, the epinephrine is reduced by half. For the donor tumescence for women, the donor tumescent anesthesia consists of 0.1% lidocaine with 1:1,000,000 epinephrine (1:500,000 epinephrine for men) made by mixing 250 mL of normal saline, 12.5 mL of 2% plain lidocaine, and 0.625 mL of 1:1000 epinephrine (1.25 mL of 1:1000 epinephrine for men). The recipient tumescence has the same concentrations but with an additional steroid component to reduce postoperative forehead edema. Because less recipient tumescence is generally used, the mixture of 0.1% lidocaine, 1:1,000,000 epinephrine (1:500,000 epinephrine for men), and 4 mg/mL of triamcinolone acetonide is made by using a mixture of 100 mL of normal saline, 5 mL of 2% plain lidocaine, 0.25 mL of 1:1000 epinephrine (0.5 mL of 1:1000 epinephrine for men), and 1 mL of 40 mg/mL of triamcinolone acetonide.

Donor Harvesting General Principles

There are 2 major methods to harvesting donor hair: FUT using a linear strip method and FUE using individual graft punch harvesting.[10] Typically, with FUE, the donor hair is shaved. In some cases, no-shave FUE can be undertaken in which individual follicles are painstakingly harvested throughout the donor area without shaving the surrounding hairs. Alternatively, a microstrip technique can be done to harvest follicles by harvesting grafts by FUE in small linear rows. The author practices the full gamut of the above FUE methods but

does not believe they make the most sense for most women who wear their hair long. For almost every woman, FUT is the preferred method of harvesting for multiple reasons. First, it is the most expedient method to harvest the hairs. Second, no shaving is required. Third, the donor hair at times can be sparse in women, and FUE over a wide area can actually further thin out the hair. Although FUE graft quality is now approaching FUT graft quality, FUT grafts are still the gold standard in terms of quality owing to the atraumatic harvest (no rotary damage) and the generous adnexa that surrounds each graft. For all of these reasons, FUT is superior to FUE for women in most cases.

When performing FUT surgery for women, there are some considerations that apply to women that may not apply as much to men. As mentioned earlier, oftentimes the temporal area is too thin to harvest hair and the entire strip must be taken from the occipital region between the mastoid prominences. For this reason, sometimes a wider strip, for example, 1.2 to 1.5 cm, must be taken to obtain enough grafts for transplantation. However, obviously if there is too much tension, then there will be poor scarring and related postoperative shock loss in the donor area. It is important to gauge how much tension can be safely handled in the donor area no matter the gender through careful manual palpation. For the novice or the individual who needs it, using the Mayer-Paul scale of laxity can be a helpful guide. In every operative case, injection of hyaluronidase above and below the strip can truly reduce total wound-closing tension and improve scar results even in patients without significant tension along the wound edge. A standard 150-unit bottle is diluted into 5 mL of saline and then equally dispersed about 1 cm above and below the wound edge approximately 10 minutes or longer before final wound closure. With greater wound tension, additional units of hyaluronidase can be used. It takes approximately 10 minutes for the surgical wound edges to relax after injection of hyaluronidase.

In most cases, women do not lose a significant amount of hair in the crown region, although they do lose some hair in the crown. For this reason, the donor incision can be placed higher in the occipital region because there is no real fear that the incision would be exposed and the transplanted hair lost with the progression of female-patterned hair loss in the crown region. This observation gives more freedom in the placement of the donor incision. The most important criterion to determine the position of the donor incision is the quality and quantity of donor hair available with the caveat that too low an incision below the occipital protuberance may lead to unfavorable scarring, that is, harvesting hair in the nuchal region. Another consideration is that sometimes women like to wear their long hair tied up in a bun in the back, and there is a minor risk of seeing an incision in the back if the donor scar heals poorly for whatever reason. Accordingly, placement of the donor incision higher up may help in camouflaging the incision when the hair is tied up and is another consideration that can be kept in mind. If there is undue tension on the wound, botulinum toxin (even 5–10 units) can be injected above and below the incision that can help with any discomfort and also possibly improve wound healing.

Recipient-Site Creation Introduction

The following sections describe specifically how to undertake recipient-site creation for the various hair loss conditions that women experience. To reiterate, these sections will not offer a step-by-step outline of how to perform hair transplant, because that would be covered by other contributors in this issue. Instead, the objective is to discuss the salient points of how hair transplantation differs in women and thereby explain to the reader the fundamental principles needed to perform superior female hair transplantation.

Besides reducing the epinephrine load, there are other important elements to reduce the extent of postoperative shock loss in women undergoing hair restoration. First, dense packing recipient sites should be avoided because doing so can predispose toward excessive hair shedding postoperatively. Also, a generous use of recipient tumescent fluid on the order of 80 to 100 mL may also heighten the odds for postoperative hair loss. In general, a more conservative amount of 20 to 50 mL is preferred depending on the size of the area to be transplanted. This method used commonly in men stands in contradistinction to donor tumescence where routinely about 150 to 250 mL is used to limit the risk of transecting the donor hair and the neurovasculature.

Female Hairline Lowering/Female Hairline Creation

This section discusses how to design recipient sites to create a female hairline that can be used in a variety of situations: a congenital high hairline, female hair loss along the hairline (**Fig. 10**), traction alopecia, hairline hair loss due to prior cosmetic surgery or trauma, male-to-female transgender hairline design, and in combination with female hair loss in other regions of the scalp. There are 2 ways to lower a congenitally high female hairline: surgical hairline advancement and hair transplantation. This section only discusses the latter method. The benefit of surgical hairline advancement is that it provides a rapid aesthetic result in a patient but it fails to address the temporal hair, which cannot be easily advanced. Oftentimes it still must be combined with hair transplant after a few months to address the temporal hair frame if the patient should so desire it.

In general, the female hairline is uniquely shaped differently than for men both in terms of its overall shape (macro hairline) and in the actual recipient sites (microhairline). When looking at the profile of an individual in the Frankfort horizontal plane, the angle from the center of the hairline to the lateral point of the hairline (at the lateral canthus) should be pointed downward in women and should never point downward in men. The shape of a female hairline is typically rounded but in actuality exhibits many different configurations, including rectangular, square, oval, circular, and hybrids of these shapes. It is suggested for the beginning surgeon to evaluate many nonbalding female hairlines to appreciate the subtle but striking differences that exist in reality. However, in most cases, a rounded design will fit most women to render a beautiful and feminine frame. It is important for the surgeon to apply artistic judgment when designing a hairline shape to provide the most attractive appearance for a particular woman. For example, if the head appears very long vertically, then a wider hairline design may make the face not appear even longer. Contrariwise, if the forehead is very broad, the hairline could be brought more inward to make the forehead look less expansive with the caveat that a narrower forehead should be balanced with width of the lower two-thirds of the face. Besides the overall shape of the hairline, another 2 components to the macrohairline involve the central widow's peak and the lateral mounds. Many

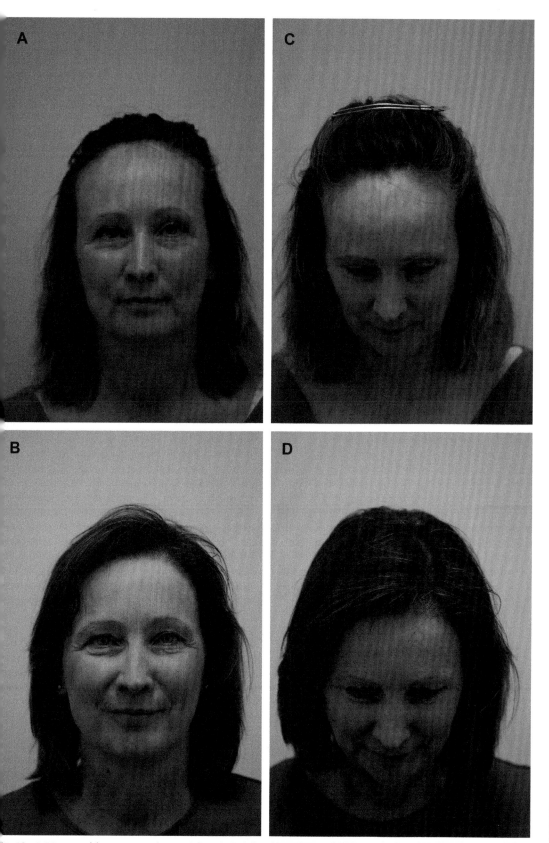

Fig. 10. A 54-year-old woman underwent female hairline lowering and is shown before (*A, C*) and 1 year after (*B, D*) hair transplant into her hairline and temples. (*Courtesy of* Dr. Samuel M. Lam.)

women exhibit a central widow's peak that also visually breaks up the linearity of the design. One or 2 rounded outcroppings of the hairline laterally can be present as well, which are termed lateral mounds and which can further soften the hairline design.

For the microhairline, that is, the recipient-site creation, typically the design involves a rotating whorl pattern that begins off center on 1 side of midline (**Fig. 11**). However, there are many variations in female hairlines, and it is imperative to study the existing hairs to determine the best design (**Fig. 12**). Again, it is worth evaluating nonbalding female hairlines to see how hairs naturally grow. One basic principle of recipient-site design is that there are no abrupt changes in angles anywhere on the scalp. Hairs gradually change angles, and it is important to mimic how nature behaves so that the result appears natural and the hair is combable. For the beginning or even the advanced surgeon, one can begin at the existing hairline and build the hairline forward, taking care not to lose the drawn hairline. Proceeding from back to front can ensure that one does not accidently run out of grafts. However, if the surgeon is confident that there will be a sufficient number of hair grafts, then it can be easier to start with the anterior hairline and work backwards to the existing hairline. It also may be helpful to draw in the radial lines on the scalp of the planned recipient-site design pattern to follow those lines during the recipient-site creation (**Fig. 13**). With coarser, straighter, and/or higher-contrast hairs that risk appearing unnatural along the hairline, a greater number of 1-hair grafts should be planned to ensure a natural-appearing result, sometimes as many as 400 to 500 grafts occupying 4 to 5 rows across the

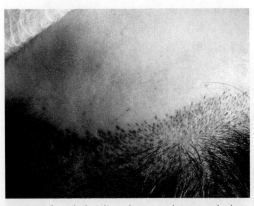

Fig. 11. A female hairline close-up photograph shows the whorl pattern starting on the left side of the scalp for a feminine-designed hairline. (*Courtesy of* Dr. Samuel M. Lam.)

entire hairline. Typically, the deeper undulations that are necessary for a male hairline with a greater number of sentinel hairs (free-floating single hairs in front of the hairline) so that the hairline appears natural are not as necessary for female hairlines. Female hairlines can appear relatively straight (not entirely straight) and appear natural. The reason for this observation is that, in men who are restoring their hairlines oftentimes the goal is to show a mild degree of natural recession, whereas in women the goal is usually (if possible) to create a strong hairline with no evidence of hair loss. Besides the difficulty of creating the rotating whorl of a female hairline, the greatest difficulty for a beginning surgeon and the number one reason a beginning surgeon should avoid undertaking female hairline re-creation is that the temple recipient sites must be placed at a very low angle vis-à-vis the scalp to appear natural. Even a slight degree of elevation of the recipient sites may appear entirely unnatural and be very difficult to correct. In addition, a right-handed surgeon may have particular difficulty creating the angles on the left temple and also have a more arduous time matching the same angles on both the right and the left sides.

If a woman is experiencing hair thinning along the hairline and needs the hairline reinforced then the surgeon should study the existing hairs to mimic their pattern when designing recipient sites. Evaluating the angle and direction of so called ghost hairs, the small residual vellus hairs left behind, can help the surgeon determine how to design the recipient-site pattern. The surgeon may be surprised at how complicated the existing female hairline pattern could in fact be: at times the hairs start by growing straight backward and then turn almost perpendicular over time to 1 side or another and then turn once again. Following this pattern in design may not only be difficult for the surgeon but also for the assistant team in charge of placing the grafts. For this reason, an operative diagram illustrating how the angles of the recipient sites were made can be helpful for the assistant team when the recipient sites veer away from a normative design or even when they do not (**Fig. 14**). If most hairs in the existing hairline are gone and only a few vellus hairs remain, then the surgeon can have a greater artistic license to design the hairline as he or she believes would be ideal for a particular patient. However, the design must always integrate with the angles of the existing hairline where the strong, terminal hairs begin because, as mentioned, there should not be any abrupt angle changes in the recipient site pattern.

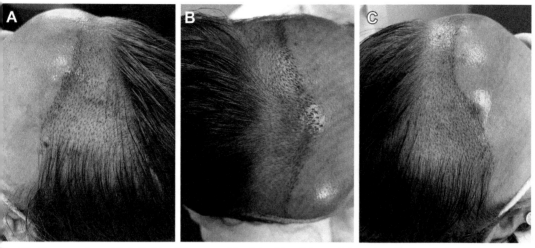

Fig. 12. Close-up views (*A*): left side, (*B*): center, (*C*): right side of the recipient sites for female hairline creation in which the recipient sites all are aimed posteriorly and downward to match the patient's existing hairs. (*Courtesy of Dr. Samuel M. Lam.*)

Restoration of Lost Hair Density

Restoring central hair density may or may not involve hairline work, because some women can lose hair density but retain the full integrity of their hairline. This section is devoted to discussing techniques in restoring central hair density. The reader is reminded to review the content in the preoperative considerations section discussing the 3 recommended patterns of L, T, and reverse L to achieve improved hair density in women by selectively targeting how they part their hair. This design strategy can be critical to maximize outcomes, especially in the face of poor donor hair density and more global hair loss demanding transplantation. Of course, if the L, T, or reverse L has been adequately transplanted, the surgeon

can then progress to other areas of secondary importance or instead tighten up the initial pattern. Another configuration is a dumbbell design (**Fig. 15**), whereby the front area is transplanted, more heavily progressing to a narrower area posteriorly (like the aforementioned Christmas-tree

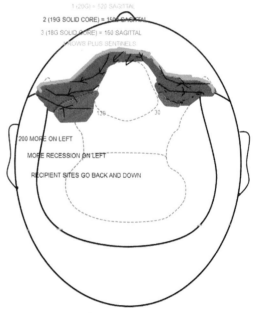

Fig. 14. Diagram (for patient featured in **Figs. 12** and 13) used as part of the operative note from the patient's electronic medical record. It is oftentimes printed out and posted in the operating room to guide the assistants during graft placement. (*Courtesy of Dr. Samuel M. Lam.*)

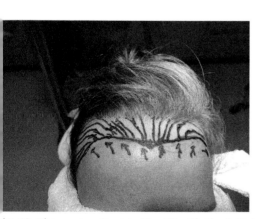

Fig. 13. The same patient in **Fig. 12** with the initial macrohairline drawn in and the radial lines that serve as guides on the design of the recipient sites. (*Courtesy of Dr. Samuel M. Lam.*)

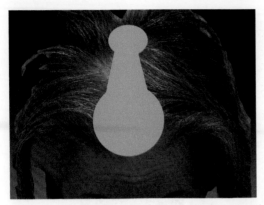

Fig. 15. A "dumbbell design" in which the central forelock is targeted principally with a tapering design progressing posteriorly to match the Christmas-tree type of hair loss and with an expansion posteriorly to accommodate the crown hair thinning that leaves a woman with a flatter appearance in the back of the head. (*Courtesy of* Dr. Samuel M. Lam.)

pattern) and then expanding again a little to cover the crown. Most women do not lose a lot of hair in the crown, but they lose the lift of hair toward the crown, rendering their hair flat in the back. This common complaint would encourage the surgeon to address a central core of hair whereby the flattening effect of the hair is remarked and to restore that area in particular. Of course, some women do lose a lot of crown hair, resembling male-patterned baldness, and the crown may need to be more extensively transplanted.

Corrective Hair Restoration Postcosmetic Surgery, for Example, Facelift, Brow Lift

Brow lifts and facelifts are relatively common reasons for loss of hair along hairline, temples, sideburn, and postauricular areas. These scars typically do well with standard transplantation methods using needles or blades, unlike linear donor strip scars that would benefit from making recipient sites with circular punch excisions. The author's success with these types of transplants could be at least partially attributed to the extensive use of regenerative medicine used in every case, namely, PRP, ACell Matristem Micromatrix (ACell, Inc, Columbia, MD, USA), liposomal ATP (Energy Delivery Solutions, Jeffersonville, KY, USA), and the storage medium of HypoThermosol (BioLife Solutions, Inc, Bothell, WA, USA), all of which improve graft survival dramatically. These methods will not be discussed in this article, but the reader is referred to the author's textbooks, video lectures, and other sources in which he recounts the detailed recipe of how he uses these important adjunctive measures for improved clinical outcomes.

Eyebrow Hair Transplant

With the trend in the past few years toward thicker eyebrows, there has been an increasing demand for eyebrow transplants. Sometimes the transplants are used to cover the poor "Groucho Marx"-style eyebrow tattoos of the past, which have fortunately given way to the more delicate and natural-appearing technique of microblading. Eyebrow hair restoration represents the highest art for a hair surgeon, and it is the most difficult to perform well. Not only is the design of the eyebrow shape and position an important dimension to master but so is the art of recipient-site creation, which is far more difficult (**Fig. 16**). The author has run a national hair course now for more than a decade, and many neophyte attendees desire to begin their career in hair restoration performing eyebrow transplant, falsely believing that this would be an easy start for them when in fact it is perhaps the single most difficult procedure to perform correctly, is the hardest to correct when done poorly, and leaves the most obvious stigma of bad hair surgery. The hairs turn in many directions, which is very hard to simulate, but the most difficult issue is ensuring that the hairs remain completely flat on the scalp because any elevation will appear unnatural. In addition, the surgical staff assisting must be of the highest caliber and possess the most extensive experience because placing grafts into eyebrow recipient sites is also very technically demanding.[11]

This section does not describe how to perform eyebrow hair transplant in a stepwise fashion because of space constraints. However, some key points are covered that have served the author well in delivering consistently excellent outcomes. Although coronal (perpendicular) recipient sites are well known to permit a recipient site that has almost no elevation, the recipient-site pattern of the eyebrow is very hard to follow when designing with coronal incisions. In addition, because the recipient sites are so flat, it is very easy to inadvertently join recipient sites, especially with coronal incisions. Parallel (sagittal) recipient sites, on the other hand, offer the 2 advantages of being able to see the designed pattern very easily and to be able to densely place recipient sites much more closely to 1 another. However, parallel sites incur the higher risk of sites that are angled too high, that is, not sufficiently flat enough to the scalp. A very slow, meticulous site creation must be undertaken, and a third bend of the needle used for site creation allows for the needle to be almost flush with the skin (**Fig. 17**). This technique can also be used when designing the low angles necessary

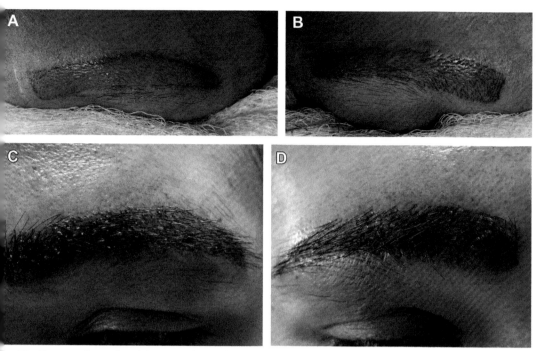

Fig. 16. Close-up views of recipient sites for eyebrow hair transplant for the left (*A*) and right (*B*) sides and immediately after graft placement for the same patient for the left (*C*) and right (*D*) sides. The perimeter of the eyebrow consists of approximately 100 1-hair sites made with a 22-gauge needle in a sagittal orientation, and the center of the eyebrow consists of approximately 250 2-hair sites made with a 21-gauge needle also in a sagittal orientation. (*Courtesy of* Dr. Samuel M. Lam.)

or temple hair transplant. In addition, because the head is round, it is important that the head be rotated as the eyebrow tail is approached to avoid the recipient sites from being angled too high. Furthermore, in the past, exclusive use of 1-hair grafts for the entire eyebrow almost always demanded a patient to return for a secondary procedure to achieve adequate hair density. Now, instead, the perimeter of the eyebrow is created with a 21-gauge needle (at times a 20 gauge in thicker-hair patients or in some African Americans) to accommodate 1-hair grafts, and the central density is created with a 20-gauge needle (at times a 19 gauge) to accommodate 2-hair grafts. Even though there is a fear that these grafts will not appear natural, they absolutely appear natural not only on casual inspection but also under close-up scrutiny. Finally, despite all efforts to create very flat recipient sites, the grafts may still appear lifted. Patients are advised to wear a snug but not tight elastic bandage around their head over the created eyebrows starting at a week postoperatively for a period of 2 to 3 weeks at night and then to resume again when the hairs begin to grow in a few months later so as to train the eyebrow hairs to grow flat. In addition, moustache wax can be used to flatten eyebrows to

help them grow flatter as needed. Patients should be given small eyebrow shears that facilitate eyebrow hair trimming and make the eyebrow hairs appear more natural than can be achieved with regular scissors.

Reconstructive Hair Transplant, for Example, Chemotherapy/Radiation, Cancer, Trauma

Hair transplant into areas of hair loss caused by chemotherapy, radiation, cancer, trauma, and so forth, can be undertaken in a similar fashion to standard hair transplant techniques. As mentioned for facelift/brow-lift scars, it is not necessary in many cases to make recipient sites with a circular punch instrument to remove the scar. However, the author's success in transplanting these types of scars where blood supply may be compromised could be partly attributed to the use of the regenerative methods outlined previously. Nevertheless, it is important to see some blood return upon pricking the area with a needle, and during recipient-site creation the surgeon should go deep enough beyond the scar to see blood flashback or the grafts may not survive well. It is always advisable to counsel the patients on the limitations of transplanting into prior scar and the possibility for additional transplant sessions as needed.

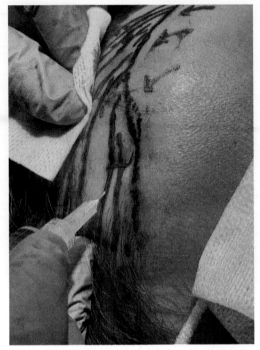

Fig. 17. To create recipient sites for an eyebrow or temple hair transplant, the angles must be very flat on the scalp. To facilitate proper site creation, there should be a third bend in the needle to allow the needle to easily lie flush. The first 2 bends of the needle serve to limit the depth of the incision and are matched to the graft length. (*Courtesy of* Dr. Samuel M. Lam.)

Obviously, dermatologic conditions like scarring alopecia represent a distinct category whereby success rates are usually very low, and disease reactivation could further compromise or destroy previously attained success.

POSTOPERATIVE CONSIDERATIONS

Postoperative care for women following hair transplant does not differ from that for men. Liposomal ATP that was used intraoperatively can be sprayed on the transplanted areas every hour while awake for the first few days until the bottle is emptied. No showering is permitted for 24 hours, and then gentle shower pressure is permitted for the first week. Minoxidil is stopped 2 days before surgery and resumed 1 week postoperatively. LLLT can be started the day after surgery. No bandages are used postoperatively. The patient applies an emollient on the transplanted area after the first week and is instructed to vigorously scrub away the remaining scabs to facilitate faster healing. Donor sutures are removed ~7 to 15 days postoperatively.

To reiterate, the most important postoperative consideration for women can be managing any postoperative hair shedding. It is important to remind the patient that if shedding occurs that should compromise their socioprofessional interactions, then the measures outlined previously, for example, creative hairstyling, use of hair fibers, or even wigs, should be used until the hairs begin to grow in and the shocked hairs return.

SUMMARY

Hair restoration in women represents an advanced topic, both medically and surgically, and should be approached cautiously by beginning hair surgeons. This article attempts to describe the full gamut of hair diseases from which women suffer and their medical and surgical remedies. Preoperatively, it is important to investigate a patient thoroughly with a complete history, physical examination, biochemical panel, and as needed, scalp biopsy. When taking a clinical history, female hair conditions can be divided into stable and unstable, with the latter being a contraindication for surgery. When performing a physical examination, female hair conditions can be divided into patchy and patterned, with the former possibly encouraging the surgeon to perform a biopsy or to elicit the aid of a dermatologist. Postoperative hair shock loss occurs in almost all women and should be counseled preoperatively and minimized by minoxidil administration; managed intraoperatively by reduced epinephrine, reduced recipient tumescence, and avoidance of dense packing; and treated postoperatively with minoxidil, creative hair styling, camouflaging hair fibers, and possibly wigs or partial hairpieces as needed. Techniques to design a natural female hairline were discussed along with caution to avoid hairline creation and eyebrow hair transplant for the beginning surgeon because the very flat angles of recipient sites can make natural results difficult to obtain for beginners. Finally, standard postoperative instructions were given that would be applicable for both genders. It is hoped that the reader gains a greater appreciation for the nuances of evaluation, counsel, medical therapy, and surgical intervention necessary when treating women for hair restoration.

DISCLOSURE

The author has nothing to disclose.

REFERENCES

1. Olsen EA. Disorders of hair growth: diagnosis and treatment. New York: McGraw-Hill Professional; 2003.

2. Lam SM, editor. Hair transplant 360: advances, techniques, business development, and global perspectives, vol. 3. Delhi (India): Jaypee Brothers Medical Publishers; 2014.

3. Unger WP, Shapiro R, editors. Hair transplantation. 4th edition. New York: Marcel Dekker; 2004.

4. Price V, Mirmirani P, editors. Cicatricial alopecia: an approach to diagnosis and management. New York: Springer; 2011.

5. Lam SM. 2nd edition. Hair transplant 360 for physicians, vol. 1. Delhi (India): Jaypee Brothers Medical Publishers; 2015.

6. Shin HS, Won CH, Lee SH, et al. Efficacy of 5% minoxidil versus combined 5% minoxidil and 0.01% tretinoin for male pattern hair loss: a randomized, double-blind, comparative clinical trial. Am J Clin Dermatol 2007;8(5):285–90.

7. Liu KH, Liu D, Chen YT, et al. Comparative effectiveness of low-level laser therapy for adult androgenic alopecia: a system review and meta-analysis of randomized controlled trials. Lasers Med Sci 2019. https://doi.org/10.1007/s10103-019-02723-6.

8. Hausauer AK, Jones DH. Evaluating the efficacy of different platelet-rich plasma regimens for management of androgenetic alopecia: a single-center, blinded, randomized clinical trial. Dermatol Surg 2018;44(9):1191–200.

9. Ablon G, Kogan S. A six-month, randomized, double-blind, placebo-controlled study evaluating the safety and efficacy of a nutraceutical supplement for promoting hair growth in women with self-perceived thinning hair. J Drugs Dermatol 2018; 17(5):558–65.

10. True RH. Strip versus FUE considerations. In: Lam SM, Williams KL, editors. Hair transplant 360: follicular unit extraction, vol. 4. Delhi (India): Jaypee Brothers Medical Publishers; 2016. p. 121–31.

11. Karamanovski Vance E. 2nd edition. Hair transplant 360 for assistants, vol. 2. Delhi (India): Jaypee Brothers Medical Publishers; 2015.

Complications with Hair Transplantation

Bahar Nadimi, MD[a,b,*]

KEYWORDS

- Complications • Hair transplant • Hair restoration • Hair

KEY POINTS

- Complications related to hair transplant surgery are usually preventable and most often caused by poor surgical planning or faulty surgical technique.
- Preoperative education and active patient participation are important for a successful postoperative course.
- Young patients are most likely to experience a planning error because of their frequent desire for aggressive restoration goals and the unpredictability of future hair loss.
- A thorough preoperative screening assessment is required to exclude patients with unrealistic goals and expectations.

INTRODUCTION

Major complications associated with well-performed and carefully planned hair transplant surgery are rare. Surgical complications are categorized as those occurring in the recipient site and those occurring in the donor site. Fortunately, complications, such as infection and bleeding, are extremely uncommon for patients undergoing hair transplantation, because the scalp has an excellent circulation that provides relative resistance to such problems. Issues associated with hair transplantation are more likely to develop from elements that are directly controlled by the surgeon or patient.[1]

Patient-related factors and patient education can also influence the occurrence of postoperative problems. Preoperative patient education is required to decrease the risk for postoperative complications. Other potential causes for hair transplant complications include patient dissatisfaction associated with body dysmorphic disorder and the unexpected loss of donor hair that may occur many years after the restoration procedure.

GENERAL COMPLICATIONS

Bleeding

Bleeding following hair transplantation can occur in the recipient and donor areas. The preoperative evaluation should screen for history of bleeding disorders and for intake of aspirin, nonsteroidal anti-inflammatory agents, vitamin E, alcohol, anabolic steroids, or other anticoagulative agents. Intraoperative recipient-site bleeding is not uncommon and can usually be reduced by injection with epinephrine-containing solutions.[2] Significant bleeding in the donor region is encountered with strip harvesting or follicular-unit extraction (FUE) following inadvertent vascular transection in the supragaleal plexus. Suture ligation best controls hemorrhage from large vessels. Coagulation is effective for sealing small vessels located in the deep tissue bed, but should be avoided for dermal bleeding because of the risk of thermal injury to the follicles. Dermal oozing is best controlled with epinephrine-containing solutions and with meticulous wound closure that firmly approximates the opposing subcutaneous edges. Patients are instructed to control postoperative oozing from

[a] Department of Otolaryngology–Head and Neck Surgery, Loyola University Medical Center, 2160 South First Avenue, Maywood, IL 60153, USA; [b] Chicago Hair Institute (Private Practice), 1S280 Summit Suite C-4, Oakbrook Terrace, IL 60181, USA
* Chicago Hair Institute, 1S280 Summit Suite C-4, Oakbrook Terrace, IL 60181.
E-mail address: drsnadimi@gmail.com

Facial Plast Surg Clin N Am 28 (2020) 225–235
https://doi.org/10.1016/j.fsc.2020.01.003

the donor sites with 10 to 15 minutes of continuous pressure. Persistent bleeding from either region requires further evaluation.

Infection

Although the incidence of infection following hair transplantation is low, localized infections can occur in the recipient- and donor-site regions. Serious infections occur in less than 1% of cases and are usually associated with poor hygiene, excessive crust formation, or a preexisting medical risk factor.[3]

Donor-site infections may be more likely following a high-tension closure secondary to the circulatory compromise associated with this situation. Excessive crust formation favors localized bacterial proliferation, which can increase the risk of infection. Recipient-site infections often present with papulopustules localized to the area, whereas donor-site infections commonly show excessive crust formation, inflammation, and light purulent discharge along the suture line. Early donor-site problems often respond well to staple and suture removal. Low-grade infections in either region tend to improve quickly with excellent wound care with removal of overlying crusts. Moist compresses and frequent shampooing are recommended to soften and dislodge adherent crusts within the recipient site and along the donor incision line. Topical antibiotic ointment is applied two times daily over any involved area to prevent additional crust formation.

Rarely a localized area in the graft site or along the incision line demonstrates fluctuance, erythema, and tenderness suggestive of abscess formation. Localized purulent fluid collections require drainage and wound care with moist gauze packs. Fluid samples should be submitted for culture and sensitivity testing to guide antimicrobial management. Although topical antibiotic ointments may suffice for managing small, well-localized inflammatory reactions, diffuse infections with surrounding erythema, edema, or tenderness generally require systemic broad-spectrum antibiotics with ideal coverage determined by final culture report.

Edema

Hairline restorations tend to generate some soft tissue edema within the forehead and surrounding areas. Occasionally, forehead edema can spread to the periorbital region. Forehead edema results from the cumulative anesthetic fluid loads injected into the recipient site and from the venous and lymphatic congestion that accompanies incising the recipient site. Patients undergoing a dense-pack or a megasession procedure are especially predisposed to edema formation. Peak facial edema usually occurs 2 to 4 days postoperatively. Patients are encouraged to rest, maintain a 45-degree head elevation, apply ice packs over the forehead region, and maintain a low-sodium diet.[4]

DONOR-SITE COMPLICATIONS

Table 1 summarizes donor-site complications.

Wide Scars

Unpredictable variations in wound healing risk the chance of a wide donor scar for some patients despite excellent surgical technique. Most patients, however, heal with a narrow scar that is easy to camouflage when proper surgical technique is carried out during donor strip harvest. Operative strategies that encourage optimal healing include the following:

- Minimize incision-line tension, particularly in the region above the mastoid process where a higher intrinsic tension may predispose some patients to wide scars
- Avoid follicular transection by performing meticulous incisions along the entire length of the donor strip
- Perform multilayered closure techniques that limit superficial tension via secure approximation of the deep fascia
- Avoid low donor incisions near the nape of the neck where scar stretching is more likely to occur[5]

Patient-related factors can also affect donor scar width, especially during the early healing phase. Patients often wish to resume exercise immediately after suture removal, at which time the increased donor-site tension that accompanies neck flexion can widen a vulnerable scar (**Fig. 1**). Patient education should emphasize the adverse consequences associated with tension-inducing forces along the donor-site incision line. Neck-flexion restrictions are recommended for 4 to 6 weeks or until the scar reveals evidence of complete maturation. Unsightly wide scars that result from technical errors or poor patient compliance may require a scar revision. Unfortunately, some wide scars may recur despite the best scar revision. Patients with recurrent widening despite careful surgical technique may require topical concealers, scalp micropigmentation, or FUE to provide effective camouflage.[1]

Cross-hatch Scars

Unsightly cross-hatch donor-site scars are possible with suture and staple wound closures

Table 1
Donor-site and recipient-site complications in hair-restoration surgery

Donor Site	Recipient Site
Wide scars	Hairline location or shape error
Cross-hatch scars	Prediction of male pattern baldness progression error
Keloid scars	Graft type error
Multiple scars	Graft placement error
Visible scars	Hypopigmentation
Donor-site depletion	Hair color mismatch
Wound dehiscence	Chronic folliculitis
Necrosis	Necrosis
Effluvium (shock-loss)	Effluvium (shock-loss)
Hypoesthesia	Ingrown hairs
Neuralgia and neuromas	Cysts
Hematoma	Low graft yield

A tight closure and pronounced edema can create a strangulation effect on the skin surface arising from tight overlying sutures or staples (**Fig. 2**). Loss of hair follicles may follow beneath each cross-hatch scar to further exacerbate the consequences of this complication. Preventive measures begin with minimizing incision-line tension through the use of conservative strip widths and layered wound-closure techniques. Patients are instructed to use frequent postoperative icing to minimize incision-line edema, and to limit neck flexion until sutures have been removed.

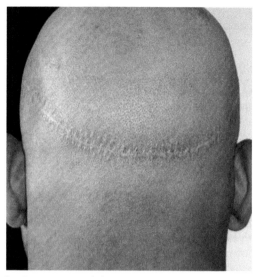

Fig. 2. Pronounced donor scar cross-hatching caused by a tight suture closure. (*From* Konior RJ. Complications in hair-restoration surgery. Facial Plast Surg Clin North Am. 2013;21(3):508; with permission.)

Keloid and Hypertrophic Scars

Donor-site keloid and hypertrophic scar formation occurs infrequently in patients without prior history of such scarring. Patients with a documented keloid tendency are discouraged from undergoing elective scalp surgery (**Fig. 3**). Proliferative scars is

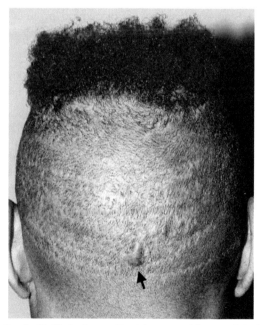

Fig. 3. Multiple donor-site strip scars with an occipital keloid scar (*arrow*). (*From* Konior RJ. Complications in hair-restoration surgery. Facial Plast Surg Clin North Am. 2013;21(3):508; with permission.)

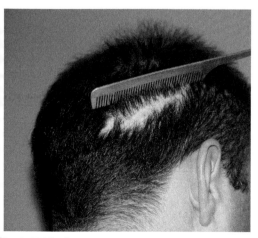

Fig. 1. Wide donor scar.

managed with intralesional injections using triamcinolone acetonide, 10 to 40 mg/mL every 4 weeks, until softening occurs.[1]

Multiple Scars

The older strategy of excising donor strips with multiple scars is rarely performed anymore. Patients often have greater difficulty camouflaging multiple donor-site scars, especially with shorter hair styles. Multiple scars scattered throughout the donor area have an adverse effect on local scalp circulation. Additionally, more donor hair must be preserved to camouflage several scars than would be needed to hide a single scar. An ideal donor-site management plan for future strip harvest procedures maintains a single scar line, accomplished by positioning a prior scar within the new donor strip or by placing it along the upper or lower edge of the newly excised strip.

Visible Scars

Visible scarring within the donor region is one of the most common complications encountered in hair transplant surgery. Surgeons who attempt to maximize graft yields through the use of aggressive donor harvesting approaches increase the risk of a long-term visible scar problems. The following methods increase this risk:

- Multiple donor incision lines scattered throughout the donor region
- Strip excisions that are placed too low in the donor region where the prevalence of scar stretching is increased
- High-density FUE graft depletion
- When strip or FUE harvests venture superiorly into donor-site fringe zones that possess a risk for future thinning

Unexpected downward migration of the donor fringe arising from progression of the balding process may expose poorly planned superior incision or extraction sites. Aggressive and repetitive donor harvests can result in "see-through" hair, which exposes donor scars even when the remaining hair is grown long. Visible scarring arising secondary to a see-through effect is difficult to correct (**Fig. 4**). In this situation, potential treatment options include donor scar grafting with body or beard hair and cosmetic tattooing.[1,6,7]

Donor-Site Depletion

Donor-site depletion is an end-stage condition where the scalp follicles are no longer available for harvest. End-stage depletion most often arises from a combination of poor surgical planning and

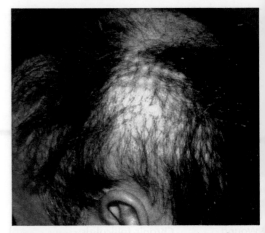

Fig. 4. Visible donor-site scarring resulting from an extremely aggressive graft-harvesting plan. (*From* Konior RJ. Complications in hair-restoration surgery. Facial Plast Surg Clin North Am. 2013;21(3):509; with permission.)

poor surgical techniques. Patients in this group commonly present with multiple problems including low graft yields, unnatural hairlines, inefficient graft distribution, and diffuse donor-site scarring.[8]

Wound Dehiscence

Donor-site wound dehiscence is extremely rare, because scalp incisions tend to heal quickly because of favorable local circulation patterns. Most surgeons remove sutures 10 to 14 days following surgery, at which time the tensile strength along the donor incision line is adequate to maintain approximation of the wound edges. Circulatory compromise, however, can delay healing and increase the risk of suture-line dehiscence. Predisposing factors, such as diabetes, smoking, a high-tension closure, suture-line infection, premature removal of sutures, and excessive early physical activity place the patient at greater risk for unexpected donor-site dehiscence.[9] This complication is best avoided by using a layered wound closure to reduce incision-line tension, avoiding early removal of sutures, and limiting any physical activities that places a distracting force on the incision line for at least 1 week following suture removal.

Necrosis

Donor-site necrosis occurs most commonly from a technical error that places excessive tension along the donor incision line. Necrosis destroys soft tissue and permanently damages follicles within the affected area (**Fig. 5**). Patients with a history of

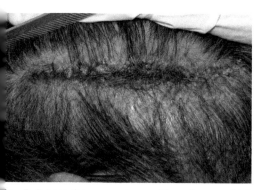

ig. 5. Donor-site necrosis resulting from a high-ension suture closure. Eschar is seen over the necrotic te in this 2-week postoperative photograph. Early ostoperative effluvium surrounds the devitalized icision site. (*From* Konior RJ. Complications in hair-estoration surgery. Facial Plast Surg Clin North Am. 013;21(3):510; with permission.)

rior scalp reduction or previous strip harvesting ay have greater intrinsic tension within their onor area, placing them at a higher risk. The pos-ibility for necrosis is increased with preexisting onditions, such as diabetes mellitus, smoking, nd donor-site scarring, and intraoperative com-lications, such as inadvertent transection of the ccipital artery.

Necrosis is best avoided by preventing exces-ive tension anywhere along the donor incision ne. The area superior to the mastoid process is articularly susceptible to a tension-related prob-em, because it often demonstrates limited laxity econdary to rigid deep scalp attachments. aution must also be exerted with wide strips at often accompany megasession donor har-ests, because these have the potential to create igh donor tension.

Once established, donor-site necrosis is managed using antibiotic ointments to provide moist occlusion to the devitalized area. Conserva-tive debridement of loose peripheral necrotic crust is performed to maintain a clean healing environ-ment. Necrotic wounds often take weeks to months to heal, and typically conclude with scar formation. The patient is encouraged to perform scalp massage for several weeks to improve local scalp laxity for potential scar revision. Serial exci-sions or tissue expansion may be required for large scars.[1]

Donor-Site Effluvium (Shock-Loss)

Minor occurrences of donor-site effluvium is com-mon. Thinning usually remains confined to a region located immediately above and below the harvest incision line. Often referred to as shock-loss, peri-incisional thinning is almost always temporary, with full recovery occurring about 3 to 4 months following surgery. Physiologic changes in the native follicle population occurring secondary to regional edema, inflammation, and localized vascular compromise along the suture line are likely contributing factors. Excessive tension along the strip incision line or inadvertent transection of major scalp vessels increase the chance of a more profound effluvium event. Fortunately, a full recovery is expected even for those with dramatic shock-loss (**Fig. 6**). Topical minoxidil is recom-mended to speed follicular recovery within the shocked zone.[10]

Neuralgias, Neuromas, and Hypoesthesia

Partial or complete nerve transection of the greater occipital, lesser occipital, or auriculotemporal nerves may occur if the incisions are made too deeply during strip harvesting. Hypoesthesia

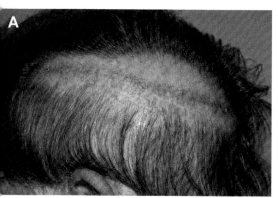
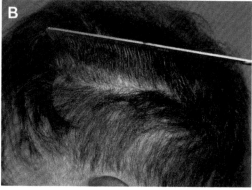

ig. 6. Donor-site shock-loss. (*A*) Dramatic donor-site effluvium. (*B*) Full recovery of donor-site effluvium at the 6-nonth postoperative photograph. (*From* Konior RJ. Complications in hair-restoration surgery. Facial Plast Surg lin North Am. 2013;21(3):511; with permission.)

localized to the innervation zone can result from accidental nerve transection. Aberrant neural healing can cause persistent scalp hyperesthesia or regional discomfort. A faulty healing response may also generate a neuroma: a tender, palpable nodule that develops from fibrous tissue proliferation surrounding the injured nerve. Treatment options for neuropathic pain or hypersensitivity arising from an injured nerve include regional infiltrations of local anesthetics and corticosteroids. Monthly injections using a mixture of triamcinolone acetonide, 10 mg/mL, diluted 2:1 with 2% lidocaine, has been recommended for this problem.[11] Extreme hyperesthesia or discomfort that resists infiltrative therapy may require referral to a neurologist for further management. Persistent pain or sensitivity arising from a palpable neuroma may require surgery to remove the mass.

Hematoma

Donor-site hematomas are rare and are usually associated with inadvertent transection of a major vessel, such as the occipital or superficial temporal arteries. Cutting too deep during strip harvesting can lacerate these vessels and, when unrecognized, may result in a donor-site hematoma. Hematomas are best avoided by limiting donor-site incision depth and carefully exploring the wound bed for evidence of vascular damage. Major vessel transections require careful suture ligation for effective control. A multilayered closure technique is preferred to eliminate any dead space that could potentially allow for a fluid collection. An active donor-site hematoma often produces pain, swelling, and localized ecchymosis. Once established, this complication is best corrected by wound exploration, suture ligation, or cauterization of actively bleeding vessels, and layered wound closure. Failure to promptly address this problem within 24 hours may increase the risk of donor-site necrosis and permanent hair loss.[12,13]

RECIPIENT-SITE COMPLICATIONS

Table 1 summarizes recipient-site complications.

Hairline Location and Shape Errors

Hairline location and shape errors occur most often in young men who prefer low and straight hairlines (**Fig. 7**). Such hairlines may appear acceptable if the balding process remains stable. Aesthetic issues of designing such a hairline may emerge if significant balding posterior to the previously set hairline occurs in the future (**Fig. 8**). Hairline design and location are determined by many factors including patient goals, available donor

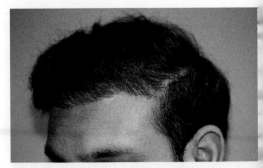

Fig. 7. A low, unnatural pluggy hairline in a young patient. Multihair grafts used at the leading edge of the frontal hairline look bulky and unnatural.

supply, and the potential for future hair loss. In general, higher hairlines that follow a gentle upward path from the central hairline to the frontotemporal recession tend to maintain a more natural appearance over time, despite aging and the ongoing progression of pattern hair loss.[1]

Prediction of Male Pattern Baldness Progression Error

A long-term planning error is most likely to occur in young patients because of the difficulty with accurately predicting the final extent of hair loss.[14] Early onset hair loss, especially during adolescence, may be a clue for future progression to a high grade pattern. Young patients who may advance to advanced hair loss patterns are especially problematic, because these individuals often have unrealistic goals for a low hairline, high density, and full scalp coverage. Aggressive restoration plans in such patients have the potential to create cosmetically disfiguring graft distributions and to deplete the donor graft supply from any future transplant surgeries.[1]

Graft Type Error

Hair transplantation has progressed from a procedure involving plugs to one that consists of individual follicular units. The primary goals of restoration focus on objectives relating to density and creating a natural appearance. Natural hair transplants are best achieved by the careful placement of meticulously dissected, individual follicular units. Unfortunately, some physicians continue to use larger minigrafts or double-unit grafts as a means of enhancing density. The frontal hairline is most prone to a detectable error of graft choice, because this is usually the most visible zone. Patients with thick skin, high-caliber hair, and a contrasting dark hair–light skin combination are especially prone to graft detectability (**Fig. 9**).

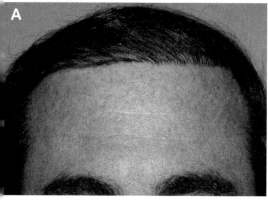
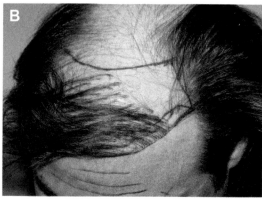

Fig. 8. (*A*) A straight and low hairline was placed on this patient 22 years earlier at 25 years of age. The patient experienced only limited frontal recession at that time and was encouraged to pursue a low hairline design. (*B*) Oblique view reveals marked progression of hair loss that occurred over 22 years following the initial restoration. The low hairline appears unbalanced, and he does not have sufficient donor supply for a complete restoration. (*From* Konior RJ. Complications in hair-restoration surgery. Facial Plast Surg Clin North Am. 2013;21(3):512; with permission.)

Small-caliber single-hair grafts should be inserted along the leading edge of the hairline to ensure a natural appearance.[1]

Graft Placement Errors

Graft placement complications commonly fall into the following categories:

1. Graft direction error (ie, wrong angle or incorrect right/left orientation)
2. Graft height error (ie, too deep or too shallow)
3. Graft rotational error

Errors relating to graft placement are completely dependent on the technical expertise of the surgical team.

Directional errors occur during preparation of the recipient sites, at which time the graft trajectory is predetermined by the path created from the blade cut into the scalp. Failure to follow the normal directional flow of hair can have adverse cosmetic consequences. Right/left directional discrepancies can create styling problems, such as difficulty establishing a natural part or hair that does not flow evenly over the recipient site (**Fig. 10**).[1]

Rotational and height errors are controlled during graft placement. Grafts placed too high result in a cobblestone appearance, whereas grafts inserted too low tend to form unattractive pits (**Fig. 11**). Extreme pitting along the frontal hairline may require FUE extraction to remove the grafts. Graft rotational errors originate from the hair shaft's natural curl, a physical characteristic that

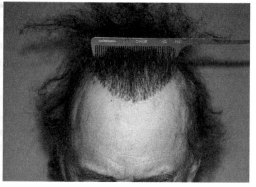

Fig. 9. Pluggy hairline/graft type error. Multihair grafts used at the leading edge of the frontal hairline look bulky and unnatural.

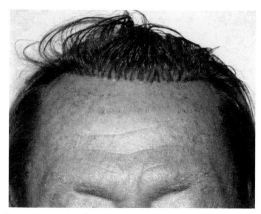

Fig. 10. Graft direction error. Improperly angled grafts placed perpendicular to the frontal scalp create an unnatural vertical wall of hair. (*From* Konior RJ. Complications in hair-restoration surgery. Facial Plast Surg Clin North Am. 2013;21(3):514; with permission.)

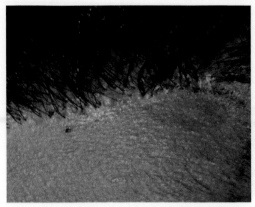

Fig. 11. Graft height error. Poor graft placement resulted in a combination of cobblestoning (too high) and pitting (too low). (*From* Konior RJ. Complications in hair-restoration surgery. Facial Plast Surg Clin North Am. 2013;21(3):514; with permission.)

imparts some element of curvature to hair. Failure to meticulously control the rotational component of graft placement so as to orient the curl appropriately can result in hairs haphazardly growing forward, upward, or with some other unnatural orientation (**Fig. 12**).[1]

Chronic Folliculitis

Chronic folliculitis is an uncommon complication of hair restoration surgery.[15] Culture and sensitivity results are typically nondiagnostic. Predisposing factors, such as poor hygiene or a concurrent dermatologic disorder, should be

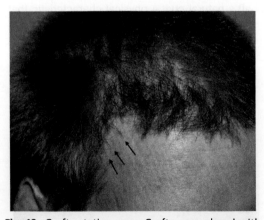

Fig. 12. Graft rotation error. Grafts were placed with the hair shaft "curl" rotated anteriorly (*arrows*), which causes transplanted hair at the temporal hairline to grow toward the forehead rather than in the natural posterior direction toward the temporal hair. (*From* Konior RJ. Complications in hair-restoration surgery. Facial Plast Surg Clin North Am. 2013;21(3):514; with permission.)

investigated for a possible etiologic source. Similar to chronic acne vulgaris, patients may demonstrate resistance to treatment. Treatment usually starts with vigorous scalp hygiene, such as daily cleansing with chlorhexidine gluconate shampoos. Topical antibiotic creams or ointments are applied over active lesions, with low-dose systemic oral antibiotics being reserved for more diffuse and resistant cases.

Cysts

Epidermal cysts originate from graft placement errors when a graft is buried beneath the recipient-site epidermal opening or when a graft is inadvertently placed over a previously placed graft.[16] Cysts in the donor site are also a potential risk with FUE, particularly following the use of a dull punch, which has the potential to push a graft deep into the donor extraction site. An epidermal cyst often presents as a tender, palpable nodule with or without surrounding erythema. Rapid resolution generally follows incision and drainage of entrapped sebaceous debris, remnant hairs, and malpositioned follicles. Localized inflammation is managed with warm moist compresses two to three times a day and application of a topical antibiotic over the affected site. Diffuse infection may necessitate the use of systemic broad-spectrum antibiotics.

Low Graft Yield

A graft yield of greater than 90% is possible with well performed, ultrarefined follicular unit transplantation.[17] A low graft survival rate is usually caused by physician-related and patient-related factors. Follicular injury that accompanies careless graft harvesting, graft preparation, or graft insertion can adversely affect graft survival. Graft desiccation is likely one of the most common preventable errors that predisposes to a low yield because the grafts typically remain vulnerable to exposure for long periods of time during the various phases of extraction, dissection, and insertion. Vascular compromise associated with such conditions as diabetes, smoking, preexisting scarring from prior trauma, previous hair restoration, or scarring alopecia can negatively affect graft yield. Extremely dense packing and large recipient-site incisions are other associated causes (**Figs. 13**). Patient-related factors that contribute to low graft yield include direct manipulation of the graft bed, such as with scratching, massaging, or aggressive shampooing.[1]

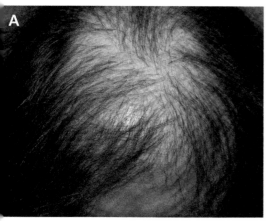
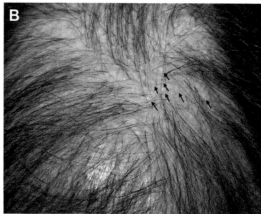

ig. 13. Low graft yield. (*A*) Patient with low yield following what was reported to be a 3000-graft session. (*B*) lose-up view of the transplant site reveals numerous hypopigmented scars (*arrows*) indicating previously placed rafts that failed to grow. (*From* Konior RJ. Complications in hair-restoration surgery. Facial Plast Surg Clin North .m. 2013;21(3):516; with permission.)

ffluvium (Shock-Loss)

tecipient-site effluvium, commonly referred to as hock-loss, occurs to some degree in most pa- ents who continue to have preexisting hair within ne transplant zone. This is characterized by shed- ing of native hair, which typically begins 2 to weeks following surgery. Most often shock-loss s temporary, but a permanent reduction in the ative hair population may occur, especially in nose hairs that are near the end of their natural fe cycle. Recovery from recipient-site effluvium enerally begins about 3 months postoperatively, round the same time as when the transplanted ollicles initiate their new growth cycle. Direct ollicular injury, regional vascular compromise,

recipient-site inflammation, and perifollicular edema increase the risk of this complication. Technical strategies that limit graft incision size, minimize the use of epinephrine infiltration, avoid dense packing, and meticulous creation of recip- ient site openings may help reduce the risk of post- operative effluvium. Topical minoxidil has been advocated to reduce the risk of effluvium and to speed the recovery of the dormant follicle population.[18]

Recipient-Site Necrosis

Recipient-site necrosis is a rare complication caused by a robust scalp blood supply (**Fig. 14**). The intraoperative appearance of persistent

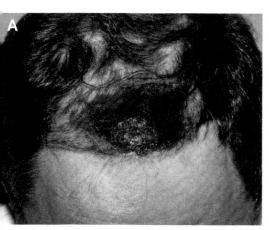
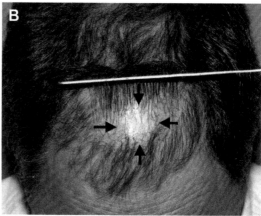

ig. 14. Recipient-site necrosis. (*A*) Two-week postoperative photograph shows dry crust densely adherent to un- erlying frontal graft zone. (*B*) Two-year postoperative photograph demonstrates cicatricial alopecia (*arrows*) ocalized to the prior necrosis zone. (*From* Konior RJ. Complications in hair-restoration surgery. Facial Plast urg Clin North Am. 2013;21(3):517; with permission.)

duskiness in the graft zone should signal immediate cessation of any additional incision or injection with epinephrine-containing solutions. Over the next few days, a compromised area typically darkens further and develops a tightly adherent superficial crust overlying the damaged soft tissue bed.

Recipient-site necrosis is a consequence of vascular compromise. Predisposing influences, such as diabetes mellitus, smoking, atrophic skin damage, preexisting recipient-site scarring, or prior scalp surgery, may increase the risk of a necrotic event. Technical factors associated with recipient-site graft placement strongly influence the potential for necrosis. Large openings, mega-sessions, dense packing, epinephrine solutions injected directly into the recipient site, and deep recipient incisions are possible contributing factors.[1]

Necrotic tissue may take weeks or months to heal. Early crust formation is best managed conservatively with moist dressings and topical antibiotics to minimize local bacterial loads and to facilitate separation of the overlying crust. A clean eschar functions as a biological dressing for the underlying wound bed, and is best managed with conservative debridement as the peripheral edges begin to separate from the scar bed below.[19] End-stage healing is marked by the emergence of cicatricial scarring.

PATIENT-RELATED COMPLICATIONS
Excessive Crusting

Grafts typically develop localized crusts over the insertion sites within 24 hours of surgical implantation. Crusts usually shed within 7 to 10 days. Crust formation normally does not create any long-term healing problems. Crust formation is best minimized with a diligent moisture-based hygiene protocol that begins immediately on completion of the procedure, at which time the recipient area is thoroughly sprayed with sterile saline solution to remove any residual blood and serum from all graft insertion sites. An early postoperative visit within 24 to 48 hours of surgery is encouraged to inspect the recipient area. Patients are advised to continue spraying frequent saline mists over the graft zone and to gently shampoo the recipient site on a daily basis until all crusts have shed. Thorough patient education as to proper spraying and shampooing methods is crucial, because some patients avoid the necessary moisturizing activities for fear of dislodging their grafts. Moist compresses, scalp soaks, and topical ointments or gels are used as needed to facilitate separation of adherent crusts.

Displaced Grafts

Patient education and compliance with postoperative instructions are vital for prevention of early postoperative graft dislodgment. Freshly placed grafts remain stable in their insertion sites only by the force of the surrounding recipient-site tissue bed and by adherence from the overlying crust. Normal wound healing requires at least 3 to 4 days to establish any significant stability between the graft and the scalp. Patients place themselves at risk during this vulnerable period with any activity that involves rubbing, combing, brushing, or striking the recipient site with a blunt or sharp force. An acutely dislodged graft is often accompanied by a sudden stream of profuse bleeding. Well-hydrated grafts are reinserted on return to the physician's office. Unfortunately, patients often return with desiccated grafts that lack viability (**Fig. 15**).[1]

Excessive Edema, Wide Scars, Low Graft Yield

The key components in minimizing patient-related complications include a comprehensive patient education program that contains clear written instructions, and frequent patient follow-up to ensure proper self-care. Inadequate postoperative care by the patient can increase the risk of edema, wide donor-site scars, low graft yield, and other potential problems.

Unexpected Progression of Hair Loss

Young patients with evidence of donor-area miniaturization are most vulnerable to an unpredictable long-term hair loss pattern. Unexpected progressions may take decades to emerge. For this reason, the surgical plan for young patients and

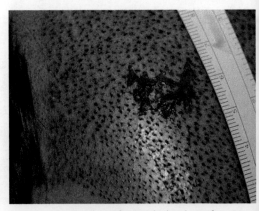

Fig. 15. Dislodged grafts. Dislodged grafts appear desiccated and devitalized. (*From* Konior RJ. Complications in hair-restoration surgery. Facial Plast Surg Clin North Am. 2013;21(3):519; with permission.)

anyone with evidence of significant donor-region miniaturization should be conservative.

Failure to Achieve Patient Expectations

At some point, most surgeons encounter an unhappy patient despite having an excellent result. This difficult scenario is best avoided by thorough preoperative patient screening, which begins with a comprehensive preoperative discussion of what is expected in terms of density, coverage, styling requirements, and any potential risks associated with the restoration process. Individuals with unrealistic goals or unreasonable expectations must be approached with caution.[1,2] Openly hostile patients with unwarranted complaints regarding prior procedures from another physician may be especially hard to please. Patients who continue to maintain unrealistic goals and expectations should be discouraged from pursuing surgery until they are willing to accept the realities of what can be accomplished. The treating physician should always remain positive, supportive, and available for future discussion.[1]

SUMMARY

Complications following hair transplantation occur infrequently with proper patient selection, a strategic operative plan, and careful execution of the transplant procedure. Patients are screened for having realistic goals and a pattern that is amenable to aesthetic restoration. A good treatment plan must factor in the potential for long-term progression of hair loss. A hair transplant should create perfectly natural-looking hair that balances the density and coverage goals agreed on by patient and surgeon. Compromising any of these key elements can increase the risk of complications and patient dissatisfaction.

DISCLOSURE

The author has nothing to disclose.

REFERENCES

1. Konior RJ. Complications in hair restoration surgery. Facial Plast Surg Clin North Am 2013;21:505–20.
2. Coleman WP III, Klein JA. Use of tumescent technique for scalp surgery and dermabrasion, and soft tissue reconstruction. J Dermatol Surg Oncol 1992;18:130–5.
3. Farjo N. Infection control and policy development in hair restoration. Hair Transplant Forum Int 2008; 18(4):141–4.
4. Nordstrom RE, Nordstrom RM. The effect of corticosteroids on postoperative edema. In: Unger WP, Nordstrom RE, editors. Hair transplantation. 2nd edition. New York: Marcel Dekker; 1988. p. 391–4.
5. Knudsen RG. The donor area. Facial Plast Surg Clin North Am 2004;12(2):233–40.
6. Pak JP, Rassman WR. Scalp micropigmentation (SMP): novel applications in hair loss. Hair Transplant Forum Int 2011;21(6):181–7.
7. Cole J. Body to scalp. In: Unger WP, Shapiro R, Unger R, et al, editors. Hair transplantation. 5th edition. London: Informa Healthcare; 2010. p. 304–6.
8. Kulaylat MN, Dayton MT. Surgical complications. In: Townsend CM, Beauchamp RD, Evers BM, et al, editors. Sabiston textbook of surgery. 18th edition. Philadelphia: Elsevier Saunders; 2008. p. 1589–623.
9. Mangubut EA. Donor area vascular damage and sequelae. In: Unger WP, Shapiro R, Unger R, et al, editors. Hair transplantation. 5th edition. London: Informa Healthcare; 2010. p. 270–1.
10. Parsley WM, Waldman MA. Management of the postoperative period. In: Unger WP, Shapiro R, Unger R, et al, editors. Hair transplantation. 5th edition. London: Informa Healthcare; 2010. p. 416–9.
11. Knudsen RG, Unger. Donor area complications. In: Unger WP, Shapiro R, Unger R, et al, editors. Hair transplantation. 5th edition. London: Informa Healthcare; 2010. p. 419–22.
12. Stough DB, Randall JK, Schauder CS. Complications in hair replacement surgery. Facial Plast Surg Clin North Am 1994;2(2):219–29.
13. Epstein JS. Different options in revision surgical hair restoration. Hair Transplant Forum Int 2010;20(3): 73–9.
14. Marritt E, Konior RJ. Patient selection, candidacy, and treatment plan for hair replacement surgery. Facial Plast Surg Clin North Am 1994;2(2):111–37.
15. Unger WP. Complications of hair transplantation. In: Unger WP, editor. Hair transplantation. 3rd edition. New York: Marcel Dekker; 1995. p. 363–74.
16. Beehner ML. Cyst formation post-transplant. Hair Transplant Forum Int 2007;17(1):30.
17. Tsilosani A. One hundred follicular units transplanted into 1 cm^2 can achieve a survival rate greater than 90%. Hair Transplant Forum Int 2009;19(1):1–7.
18. True RH, Dorin RJ. A protocol to prevent shock loss. Hair Transplant Forum Int 2005;15(6):197.
19. Nusbaum BP, Nusbaum AG. Recipient area complications. In: Unger WP, Shapiro R, Unger R, et al, editors. Hair transplantation. 5th edition. London: Informa Healthcare; 2010. p. 422–4.

Beard Hair Transplantation

Anthony Bared, MD*

KEYWORDS

- Hair restoration • Beard hair transplantation • Modern techniques • Surgery

KEY POINTS

- In the field of hair restoration, there has been a significant increase in demand with patients for facial hair transplantation procedures.
- Modern techniques in hair transplantation allow for facial hair transplantation and for the attainment of natural-appearing results.
- Facial hair transplantation is a subspecialty within hair restoration with many gratifying benefits for the patients as well as for the hair restoration surgeon.
- Adapting these advanced techniques into a hair restoration practice allows a surgeon to offer their patients these procedures and provides an expanded artistic element to a hair restoration surgeon's practice.
- In this article, hair restoration surgeons learn how to best select a candidate for beard hair transplantation, fine tune the technical and surgical aspects of the procedures, become aware of potential pitfalls, and learn how to best prevent and handle complications of these procedures.

In the field of hair restoration, there has been a significant increase in demand with patients for facial hair transplantation procedures. Modern techniques in hair transplantation allow for facial hair transplantation and for the attainment of natural-appearing results. Patients are seeking fuller beards in ever-increasing numbers because of social, fashion, and cultural trends. Pick up any of the latest fashion magazines or watch sporting events and you see models and athletes with full beards. Facial hair transplantation is a subspecialty within hair restoration with many gratifying benefits for the patients as well as for the hair restoration surgeon. Adapting these advanced techniques into a hair restoration practice allows a surgeon to offer their patients these procedures and provides an expanded artistic element to a hair restoration surgeon's practice. In this article, hair restoration surgeons learn how to best select a candidate for beard hair transplantation, fine tune the technical and surgical aspects of the procedures, become aware of potential pitfalls, and learn how to best prevent and handle complications of these procedures.

PATIENT CANDIDACY AND CONSULTATION

Patients for facial hair transplantation typically present with a rather specific idea of how they want their facial hair to appear. Most patients seeking facial hair restoration are men with a genetic paucity of facial hair. Other reasons for patients seeking facial hair restoration are for poorly thought-out prior laser hair removal, scarring, burn, or cleft lip repair (**Fig. 1**). Another small group is female-to-male transgender patients seeking a more masculine appearance. It is common for the patient presenting for beard hair restoration to bring with them photographs of their "goal" beard shape and density. A patient's goals may vary from increasing the density of an existing beard while maintaining the same shape, to transplanting full beards where very few hairs exist. The design and density of the beard may be limited by the quality and quantity of the donor area. Transplantation of full beards requires a large amount of grafts, and patients are always made aware of the possibility of undergoing secondary procedures after around 1 year if further density is

Private Practice, Miami, FL, USA
* 6280 Sunset Drive, Suite 504, Miami, FL 33143.
E-mail address: abared@dranthonybared.com

Facial Plast Surg Clin N Am 28 (2020) 237–241
https://doi.org/10.1016/j.fsc.2020.01.010
1064-7406/20/© 2020 Elsevier Inc. All rights reserved.

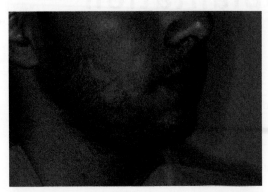

Fig. 1. Patient with acne scarring presenting for facial hair restoration to help camouflage scars. (*From* Bared A. What's new in facial hair transplantation?: effective techniques for beard and eyebrow transplantation. Facial Plast Surg Clin North Am. 2019;27(3):380; with permission.)

desired. The hair restoration surgeon needs to guide the patient as to what can be realistically achieved through a procedure. Limitations as to the extent of the height of the cheek beard hair or the coverage of the chin/goatee region are made aware to the patient. Depending on the exact design and density, graft counts can range from 250 to 300 grafts to each sideburn, 400 to 800 grafts to the mustache and goatee, and 300 to 500 grafts per cheek. These numbers can vary based on the preexisting hair, design, and thickness of the donor hair. It must be made clear that these grafts, once transplanted, will no longer be available for use in the scalp in the future if male pattern hair loss is to develop.

It is important for the hair restoration surgeon, starting in beard hair transplantation, to have an appreciation for the various levels of complexity certain beard designs present. The novice surgeon should ideally start with smaller cases and transplanting within areas of the beard that pose less of a challenge. The most challenging areas of a beard to create density are those of the central face: mustache, goatee, and the connection of the mustache to the goatee. The cases that pose the greatest challenge are those whereby the patient has little to no hair in these areas. It is more prudent for the novice surgeon to commence with cases whereby patients may have existing hair in these areas whereby the main goal is that of increasing density. It is less challenging to create density in the cheek beard than to create density in the central face. It is particularly very challenging to create density in the region connecting the mustache to the goatee. Patients need to be made aware of these limitations to the creation of density to the mustache and goatee region so proper expectations are met.

Donor hair analysis as in any other area of hair restoration is imperative to the preoperative planning. Patients with thick, dark, and very straight donor hair pose the greatest challenge in facial hair restoration. Patients with these donor hair characteristics are more at risk of taking a more unnatural appearance. It is best to start with smaller-sized cases in patients with these donor hair characteristics until one gains the experience needed in facial hair transplantation (**Fig. 2**).

With refinements in follicular unit extraction (FUE), most patients elect to have the procedure performed in this manner so as to avoid a linear scar, allowing them to maintain a short hairstyle.[1,] FUE has largely replaced the traditional strip donor extractions for beard transplantation.[3] Regardless of the donor technique used, patients are made aware of the potential limitations of the donor hair quantity and therefore "size" and density of the beard that can be achieved through solely procedure. Scalp hair transplants to the face have a very high regrowth percentage, and if properly performed, patients can achieve a very natural outcome.

PREOPERATIVE PLANNING

There is no ideal facial hair pattern, and there are many differences among different ethnic groups. As mentioned, most patients have a specific idea of the design they wish for their facial hair. On the day of the procedure, the patient is met in the preoperative suite. Using the patient's guidelines, the areas to be transplanted are marked out using a surgical marking pen with the patient in a seated position. The markings are checked for symmetry between the 2 sides. Measurements are used to help ensure symmetry. Areas where symmetry are most attended to are in the width of each sideburn, the line of curvature connecting the sideburn to the cheek beard, the level at which the cheek beard connects with the mustache, and the width of the connection between the mustache and the goatee. Patients are shown the markings in a mirror, because the 2-dimensional perspective provided by a mirror, which is what the patient sees in a mirror, is different than what the surgeon sees in direct 3-dimensions. As previously discussed with the patient during the consultation, limitations may exist as to how high the cheek beard hair may extend, for instance. If there needed, alterations are made according to patient desires.

The 1 area of caution in patients with thick or dark hair is the area immediately inferior to the lower lip, referred to as the "soul patch" area and the chin mound. Particularly in patients with thick

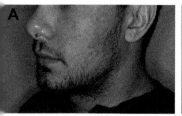 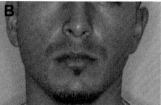 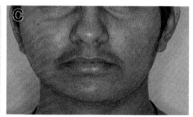

Fig. 2. Patients with increasing complexity for facial hair restoration. (*A*) Least challenging presentation of a patient with patchiness to the beard hair. (*B*) Slightly more challenging presentation of a patient with good density of the mustache but seeking to connect the mustache with the goatee. (*C*) Most challenging presentation of a patient with little to no facial hair seeking beard transplantation. ([*C*] *From* Bared A. What's new in facial hair transplantation?: effective techniques for beard and eyebrow transplantation. Facial Plast Surg Clin North Am. 2019;27(3):380; with permission.)

and dark hairs, this area is susceptible to bump formation at each graft site. Because of the risk of bump formation, this area is avoided or a few "test" grafts are placed in this area at the time of the initial procedure. If no bumps form after months, then further grafting can be done to this area.

SURGICAL PROCEDURE

Nearly all patients seeking facial hair restoration elect to have their procedure via the FUE technique in order to avoid a linear scar. In these cases, the donor area is shaved, and patients are placed in a supine position. A handheld drill with the smallest possible drill size avoiding graft transection is used for the extractions. The donor area consists of the occiput only in smaller cases and extends into the parietal scalp for larger cases. Graft extractions are evenly distributed throughout the donor area to avoid areas of focal alopecia. Once the extractions have been completed from the occipital area, the patient is then turned to lie in the supine position. Follicular units used are those of 1-, 2-, and 3-hair grafts.[5] In cases of patients with thick and dark donor hairs, the 3-hair grafts are divided into single- and 2-hair grafts.

Local anesthesia is then applied to the face, starting in each sideburn and cheek area. The area around the mouth is not anesthetized at this point, but rather the area around the mouth is typically worked on after the patient has eaten lunch. The recipient sites in the sideburn and cheek area are made first. The smallest possible recipient sites are made using 0.6-, 0.7-, or 0.8-mm slits. The 1-, 2-, and (if used) 3-hair grafts are tested to ensure size compatibility with the recipient sites. In the periphery of the sideburns, 1-hair grafts are used while 2-hair grafts can be placed in the central aspect of the sideburn to allow for more density (**Fig. 3**). Countertraction

is provided by the nondominant hand and an assistant, while making the incisions. The key aesthetic step is to make the incisions at an ultra-acute angle to the skin, with the direction of the incisions determined by either existing surrounding hairs or the fine "peach fuzz" of the face. This being said, the direction of growth is generally downward, but more centrally closer to the mouth/goatee region can be somewhat anterior (**Fig. 4**). In the cheek area, 3-hair grafts are sometimes used in the central beard in patients with finer hair to allow for the achievement of greater density without a compromise of naturalness. If further grafts are needed, they are extracted at this time from the parietal scalp. The patient's head is slightly turned, allowing for the simultaneous extraction of grafts from the parietal area and the placement of grafts in the ipsilateral cheek and sideburn.

After the patient is given lunch, the area around the mouth is then anesthetized. Infraorbital and mental nerve blocks are used to provide initial anesthesia. The goatee and mustache area anesthesia is then reinforced with field subdermal local anesthesia complemented by epi 1:50,000 to minimize bleeding. Incisions in the goatee and mustache area are then made. On the mustache, hairs will grow slightly laterally and then transition downward along the goatee. As previously mentioned, patients need to be made aware of the difficulty in creating density along the entire mustache, particularly centrally within the "cupid's bow." The creation of density in this area is difficult owing to the undulations created by the upper lip's "cupid's bow" area. It is also important to maintain as acute of an angle as possible in this central area of the upper lip because grafts have a tendency to grow straight outward in nonacute angles. The transition from the mustache to the goatee is an important area for the creation of density, which is usually created by the maximal dense packing of 2-hair grafts.

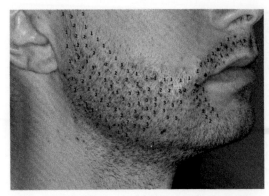

Fig. 3. The distribution of follicle graft sizes. (*From* Bared A. What's new in facial hair transplantation?: effective techniques for beard and eyebrow transplantation. Facial Plast Surg Clin North Am. 2019;27(3):381; with permission.)

The grafts are placed into the recipient using jeweler's forceps. Countertraction splaying the incision sites open with the nondominant hand helps in the placement of the grafts given the laxity of facial skin. The importance of having experienced assistants for this process is critical, because they need to understand the "pattern" of graft distribution as created by the surgeon. Toward the conclusion of the case, the patient is given a mirror before all grafts are placed. Given that the immediate results closely replicate the final results, it is helpful for the patient to view their beard in order to assess the design and density of the grafts. This step allows for feedback, fine-tuning, and alteration before the conclusion of the case (**Fig. 5**).

POTENTIAL COMPLICATIONS AND THEIR MANAGEMENT

Hairs can grow out perpendicularly, giving the beard an unnatural appearance. The area of the face where improper angulation poses the greatest challenge is in the mustache, particularly in patients with very straight hair. To avoid improper angulation, it is helpful to use the smallest possible incision at a very acute angle. It is helpful to use a longer blade so as to allow it to lay flat across the skin, permitting a sharply acute angle. If needed, the perpendicular hair grafts can be removed via the FUE technique, and the resulting hole is left to heal by secondary intention.

Tiny bumps can form in the soul patch and chin mound areas at the site of the transplanted grafts. The cause for the formation of these bumps is not known; however, this is mostly seen in patients with thick, dark hairs. Patients of Asian ethnicity, particularly those with dark thick hairs, are the most challenging on whom to avoid complications both in this bump formation and also in achieving naturalness because of the difficulty in getting the grafts to look natural, particularly in angulation. As mentioned, with patients of Asian descent, the less-experienced surgeon is strongly encouraged to proceed conservatively, with the primary use of all single-hair grafts and smaller number of grafts until proficiency is achieved. As the hair grows in this soul patch and chin mound area, a small bump can form where the hair exits the skin. For this reason, if a patient desires hair in these regions, a small "test" procedure can be performed at the time of the initial procedure. If in 6 to 8 months, no bumps have formed, then further hair can be transplanted.[6]

POSTOPERATIVE MANAGEMENT

Patients are told to keep the face dry for the first 5 days after the procedure; this allows for the grafts to set properly, helping assure the

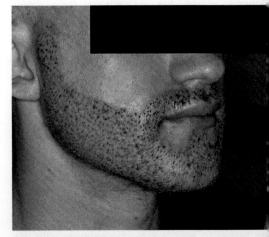

Fig. 5. Immediate postoperative results. (*From* Bared A. What's new in facial hair transplantation?: effective techniques for beard and eyebrow transplantation. Facial Plast Surg Clin North Am. 2019;27(3):381; with permission.)

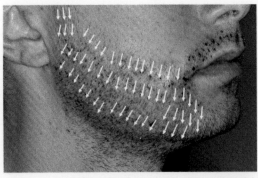

Fig. 4. The direction of hair growth in most beards.

maintenance of proper angulation. Topical antibiotic ointment is applied to the donor area. Patents are then to wet the face on the sixth ostoperative day with soap and water, starting o remove the dried blood and crusts. Shaving is ermitted after 10 days.

Pinkness to the face can be present after the rocedure and usually resolves after a few weeks. n patients with very light complexion, this pinkess can persist for longer periods. The author as found that the oral antihistamine diphenhydraine taken at night before bedtime can help educe this pinkness. Hair regrowth usually starts round 4 to 6 months. The transplanted hair can e treated as any other facial hair and allowed to row out or be shaved. Although most patients re satisfied with the initial density from 1 procedre, a secondary, touch-up procedure can be perormed after 1 year to create further density.

UMMARY

he performance of beard hair transplantation is a ery rewarding subspecialty within hair restoration /ith a high patient satisfaction rate. It provides an immediate satisfaction" for patients because they re at least able to see the shape of their future eard and foresee how their beard will appear

when the hair grafts regrow. For the hair restoration surgeon, it allows an artistic element, which can be limited in other aspects of hair restoration surgery.

DISCLOSURE

The author has nothing to disclose.

REFERENCES

1. Rassman WR, Berstein RM, McClellan R, et al. Follicular unit extraction: minimally invasive surgery for hair transplantation. Dermatol Surg 2002;28:720–8.
2. Harris J. Conventional FUE in hair transplantation. In: Unger W, Shapiro R, Unger R, editors. Hair transplantation. 5th edition; 2001. p. 291–6.
3. Donor area harvesting. Unger W, Shapiro R, Unger R, et al. Hair transplantation. 5th edition. New York: Informa Healthcare; 2011. p. 247–90.
4. Gandelman M, Epstein JS. Reconstruction of the sideburn, moustache, and beard. Facial Plast Surg Clin North Am 2004;12:253–61.
5. Bernstein RM, Rassman WR. International Journal of Aesthetic and Restorative Surgery 1995;3(2):119–32.
6. Epstein JS. Hair restoration to eyebrows, beard, sideburns, and eyelashes. Facial Plast Surg Clin North Am 2013;21:457–67.

Moving?

Make sure your subscription moves with you!

To notify us of your new address, find your **Clinics Account Number** (located on your mailing label above your name), and contact customer service at:

Email: journalscustomerservice-usa@elsevier.com

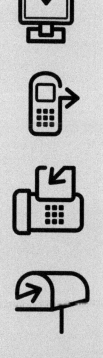

800-654-2452 (subscribers in the U.S. & Canada)
314-447-8871 (subscribers outside of the U.S. & Canada)

Fax number: 314-447-8029

Elsevier Health Sciences Division
Subscription Customer Service
3251 Riverport Lane
Maryland Heights, MO 63043

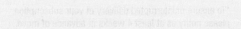

Printed and bound by CPI Group (UK) Ltd, Croydon, CR0 4YY

08/05/2025

01864746-0012